LIES
MY DOCTOR TOLD ME

Medical Myths That
Can Harm Your Health

Ken D. Berry, MD, FAAFP

VICTORY BELT PUBLISHING INC.
Las Vegas

ISBN-13: 978-1-628603-78-1

Cover Design by Justin-Aaron Velasco
Interior Design by Elita San Juan

TC 0319

To my amazing, beautiful wife, Neisha;
my children, Jonathon, Madison,
Morgan, and Abby Grace; and
my granddaughter, Adeline Virginia.
You all are my saving grace
and my inspiration.

My Generous Patrons

Dennis Frazier

Chris Bair
Shannon Clemons
John Coffman
John Cronin
LeaAnn Espat

Beverly Fuller, RN
Rumi Kollaus
Angelina Margaret
Jeff Provost
P. (Rocky) Rauchwald

Doyle Rodgers, Jr.
Joe Williams

Ada
Lou Adkins
Kay Allen
Sandra Amlong
Betsy Andrus
Brian and Donna
 Backman
Shannon Baker
Wanda M. Bedard
Sam Billingsley
Cathy Billiter
Marty and Suzanne
 Booth
John Boyles
Tonya Bozeman
Nick Brien
Lori Brubaker

Sandi Burch
Peter Burger
John Cave
Vince and Rachel
Charfauros
Elizabeth Clawson
Noah David Clifton II
Marie Cluett
Belinda Cochran
Jane Coldsnow
Cheryl Corbin
Donna M. Couch
Country Fried Zen
Holly Dahl
Robyn Davis
Catharine R. Davis
Jaclyn Dougherty

Pat Dugar
Jan Jackson Ensor
Alexis Fama
Rebecca Flake
Carl Franklin
Tia Gentry
Jill Godbout
Brenda (Bree) Goodwin
Mark T. Grace
Judy Gravenhorst
Zachery C. Gray
Gregory Grennier
Julie and Alan Guenther
Susie Hammond
Jennifer Harris
Sherri Harris
Pam Hawkins

Robin Hill
Pat Holt
Michele Holz
Helene Hopkins
Angel Hopkins
James Huskey
Sandy Irvin
Cara Jackson
Chad Jacobs
Terra Jacobus
Terri Jennings
Jazmin Jimenez
Jaynell Jordan
Katie Kavanaugh
Caresa Kelemen
Amy Knox
Deirdre Kohley

Laurie Kor
Stacy Kuhl-Cash
Marlene La Ban
Lory Lahtinen
Julie Langley
Debbie Latt
Daniele and Jay Latzman
Bobbie Robbins Leab
Kathleen Leander
Sarah Lefebvre
Samantha Lewer
Amanda Little
Randal Lovvorn
Tamara McCauley, MSN, RN
Nikki McLaughlin
Carol R. Medders
Darla Meeks

Bruce Meltzer
Stephanie Merrill
Alice Micka
Amanda Murray
Linda S. Napier
Gale Ory
Phyllis Parks
Dana Patterson
Scott Payton
Kevin Perrin
Danica Philstetler
Sue Piller
Jennilyn Pittman
Kimberley McCavitt Plomp
Joy Postell
Melissa Prestangen
Wayne Prince

Roxanne Provencher
Steven J. Provencher
Paula Ransdell
Melanie Reza
Julie Robinson
Mary Rogers
Betty J. Russell
Melissa Scarborough
Paul Schwartz
Rebecca Scribner, RN
Thomas Seest
Frederic Shry
Michael Silverman
Niki Simko
Melody C. Skelton
Nanci Smith
Molly Smithey
Gary Snyder

Christina Stones
Anthony Storino
Susan Summerville
Diann Taylor
Patty L. Terry
Shannon Timmons
Jessica Viker
Terry Vinson
Sandi Waggoner
Bret Watkins
Cheryl Werrbach
Stella White
Amanda Willis
David Wills
Christine L. Wilson
Kris Young
Carol Zlatovich

Erik Aamodt
Joseph R. Abate
Nur Abdullah
Valeria Adam
Inga Ãlafs
Maria Alexander
Shannon Alford
Deborah Allain
Brian Allen
April Allen
Brent Alley
Lena Allsup-Garland
Mary Anderson
Linda Anderson
Marsha Andrews
Lee Andrus

Ann
Lynn Anthony
Janette Aragon
Rhonda Arellano
Jessica Armer
Cernice Armstrong
Cyndi Arnold
Melanie Ashton
Reshma Asrani
Linda B.
Josh Baal
Ximena Backer
Marc Bailey
Robert P. Bailey
Nancy Baisinger
Annie Bakaleinikoff
Julie Baldi

Katie Baldwin
Terry and Jenn Baptista
Jason Barden
Holli Baughman
Stephanie Beard
John C. Beckman
Tricia Behmardi
Connie Bender
Jackie Bentz
Janet Berkman
Diana L. Bertapelle
Peg Beuoy
Kathy H. Bevard
Deb Biernacki
Krista and Pete Bifano
Ashley Binford
Lynne Blair

Ann D. Blais
Lori Blakley
LaVera Blanco
Brenda Block
Wynette Bloom
Yvette Blythe
Leita J. B-Newman
Barbara Bragole
Jennifer Brechbill
Debora Briggs
Belinda D. Broussard

Rena Brown

Scott Brown

Michael Brown

Melaine Brown

Lisa Brown

Lisa K. Brown

Sue Brown

Sara Brown

Anna Brown

Karen Brown

Holly Brown

Vesta Brown

David Browne

Kirstyn Bruno

Tony Bruscino

Chris Buchanan

Angie Bullock

Jamie Burchett

Daniel Burejsza

Suzanna Burgess

David Burke

Paulette J. Burkhart

Sara C. Globis

Jim Cadena

Frank Callahan, RN

Cindy J. Callaway

Robert Calvo

Scott Campbell

Laura Campbell

Robert M. Cape

Michael Capps

Theresa Cargo

Rene Carlson

Lynn Carnes

Laura Carr

Jess Carter

Annette Cartwright

Joyce Z. Casey

Clint Cason

Joe Cassell

Lori Chamberland

Kathy Chang

John Checki

Jeannine Cheever

Chickas5Homestead

Rob Christensen

Christy

Susan Clampitt

Paul Clark

John Clayburn

Ginger Clayton

Marcus Clemmons

Melvis Click

Cindy Clifton

Carmen H. Coates

Jack Conway

Tina Cooper

Peggy Corbett

Meredith Cornelius

Melissa Costa

Jason Cotney

Jada Cox

Patti Craft

Credit Liberation

Casey Crisler

Julia Crissey

Brandi Cronen

Jan Cropper

Randy A. Cross

Cassie Cullinan

Shelly M. Culp

Joan Curley

Daconda

Ann Daniells

Anita L. Daniels

Darth Keto

Ruth David

Debbie Davis

Dave Davis

Michael A. Davis, Jr.

Tammy Day

Ann P. Denslow

Tad Denton

Jim DePaul

Steven Depuy

Marcy DeShong

Kristin DiGennaro

Jeff and Julie Dinsdale

Joanne Dispennette

Joann L. Dixon

Sue Dodd

Chris Doherty

Pat L. Donald

Margaret T. Donovan

Angela Doucette

Beverly Downs

Mary J. Drake

James Dunbar

Renee K. Dunn

Katherine Durham

Gloria East

Tammy Eckard

Ursula Eissner

Theresa Elliott

Deb Elliott-Black

Cheryl A. Ellis

Tammy Ellison

Debbie England

KevenE. Entzel

Kimberly Eucker

Jackie Fagan

Donna Fagan

Amberly Farber

Chaka Fennell

Deborah Fennell

Nora Fernandez

Sue Ferrier

Courtney Fitzgerald

A. and Nora Fontana

Alicia Fontenot

Laura Foote

Suzee Fox

Nich. Francescutti

Tammy A. Franks

Darlene Frybarger

Brenda Gafford

Lisa Gardner

Lori G. R. Garthwaite

Jeff Geisler

Katie Gibbons

Lisa Gimber

Suzanne Glapion

Jacqueline Glasgow

Michelle Goldsmith

Susie Gonzalez

Roy Goodwin

Michael (Mike) Goril

Missy Gorman

Caitlin Gosling

Roxanne Gowin

Glenn Graham

Karen Grandfield

Kathleen Grant

Lisa T. Gray

Doug Green

Andrea Green

Joan Green

Jeremy Greer

Melanie Griffith

David Guenthner

Chris and Anna Guidroz

Mark Guinn

Brian H.

Pamela Hack

Joe B. Hackney

Beth Hahn

Donald Hallenbeck

Melinda Hamilton

Keith Hamilton

Leah Hansen

Nykol Happy

Monika Hardy

Melissa Hargrove

Sara M. Harned

Dianne Harris

Leslie Harris

Sandra Harris

Ted Harris

Jenny Hartshorn

Nathaniel Hatten

Kyle Hausrath

Lisa K. Hayes

Mariane J. Hayes

April R. Haynes

Robert Helveston

Kymberli Hemberger

Laura Hendrix

Kerry Hennessey

Debbie Hernandez

Deborah Herren

Georgia Herring

Barbara Hester

Yvette Hicks

Marla R. Hilliard

Peggy Hinman

Linda Hoffer

Pat Hoffman

Lori Hoke

Shelly Holladay

Terry Holt

Keith Homel

Samuel C. Hood

Maricris Hopkins

Ann Hotchkiss

Tom Houde

Denise L. Howard

Donald A. Huettl

Kayla Huff

A. J. Hulsey

Leanne Hunt

Susan Hunt

Charleen Hurley

Sharron Huss

Kiera Huybers

Brenda H. Ireland

Carol Iselin

Jared James

Chris Jantzen

Jeania

Lori D. Jekelis

Jennifer and David

Shirley Jezek

Lori D. Jibreen

Jennifer Jiles-Davis

Sonja Jimenez

John

Richard Johnson

Debbie Johnson

James C. Johnson

Anna Johnson

Jerrold J. Johnson

Greg Johnson

Courtney L. Johnson

Emily Johnston

Rhonda Jones

Robin Jones

Joyful Keto Life

William Judkins

DeLorie Juhasz

Deborah J-Williams

Molly Kavanagh

Steven Kelley

Robin Kendrick

Licia Kennedy

Susan Kerby

Alex Kerkstra

Sarah King

Deb King

Jen King, RN

John Kistler

Patti Kitzman

Stuart Klausner

Susyn Klein

Patricia Knigge

Christina A. Knowles

Nadine Knowles

Wendy Knuckles

Elaina Kohlhauser

Barbara Kotila

Randy Kramer

Kathi Kramer

Jim Kuder

Philip Kulp

Judith Labella

Kaleigh Laleman

Dawn Lamb

Stacy Lamb, Rmt

Sharon Lambeth

Nancie Lamson

Renee Langford

Mark A. Lantz

Tammie LaRue

Kalia Lastra

Tina Lauderman

Laura

Tammy LeClerc

Kristal Lee

Happy Lee

Eva Leonard

Prissy Leonard

Scott J. LePage

Faith L-Heidtman

Ken Lien

Amanda Lilienthal

Linda

Jerry Little

Patricia O. Loewen

Miche. Loewenstein

Thomas Lorenc

Nic Love

Judy Lowrance

Margo B. Lucas

Dana Luce

Scott Luckman

Jo (Joette) Lutrick

Kate Lutz

Janis Weber Lutz

Vicki Lutzen

Alicia M.

Marilyn MacFarland

Rebecca Mack

Patricia Magoon

Jay Magruder

Meg Magruder

Lisa Maher-Fly

Cindy Maimone

B. J. Malecha

Leslie Malloy

Roxanne Mansfield

Gregory Manzi

Maree.Rose

Sam Markwell

Kimberly Marquardt

Ericka Marsh

Laurie Marshall

Judith Martinez

April Maselli

Toye A. Mason

Anthony Masseur

Cindy Masters

Debbie Mattatall

Jason Mays

Bob McCabe

Jodi McCann

Kim McClanahan

Daniel J. McDowell

Steve McDowell

Sonya McElreath

Steph McGarrigle

Dana McGuinness

Christine McGuire

Angie McKee

Caren McKeon

Michelle McKuhen

Renee McMahon

Brigida McRae

Linda Meacham

Sharon Meck

David R. Meek

Deborah Meggison

Melissa

Margarita Messinger

Rick Messner

Michell

Amber Miller

Susan Miller

Susan Mills

Pamela Mills, MSN

Leah D. Miranda

Miss Mud Monkey

Darlene Mobley

Debbie Mogg

Molly

Christine Montano

Gavin Moore

Imogene Moore

Brittany Moose

Isael Sotelo Morales

Vicki Morgan

Jan Morgan

J. R. Moritz

Deborah L. Morrison

Shaun Morse

Suzanne E. Moseley

Patricia Moya

Cindy Mrva

Charles Muldoon

Michelle Mullins

Sandra Mullins

Andrea F. Murdock

Debbie Musselli

Lynn Musselman

Frank Myers

Jeanne Myers

MyPersKetoCoach

Patricia Nally

Suzanne Nally

Holly Ann Neeley

Alan Neff

Michele Nelson

Diana Neumann

Janet Newbill

Karla Nichols

Teresa B. Nieves

Ann and Len Niggemann

Dale Leigh Noll

Janis L. Nordmeyer

Janette O'Neil

Jodie Olson

Cathy Olson

Patricio Ortiz

Yassine Ouarzazi

Terici K. Owens

Becky Padilla

PaleoBarbie

Tamara Palmer

Mari Palmer

Tom Pape, Jr.

Kirsten Pataky

Jeffrey I. Patrick

Wanda Payne

Ronald Pearson

Kristie Peck

David Peet

Sherry Peiffer

Melanie Pendleton

Preston D. People

Norma Perry

Kathy Pesek

Peggy S. Peters

Mary Petersdorf

Eva Evans Phillips

Kathy Phillips

Amber Piersee

April Pinkston

Justine Piper

Sue Piringer

Linda Pittenger

Demetria Plevritis

Tish Pollock

Stacy M. Poor

Michael Poss

Daniel Potter

Jackie Prather

Gay Preator

Pauline Preston

Bill Priday

J. Randy Principe

Rhonda Prokupek

Greg Provost

Anne Quinlan

Elizabeth T. Raimo

Dawn Rangel

William M. Ransom

Christy Rath

Warren L. Ratliff

Vickie Ray

Greg Reeser

Kimberly Rhodes

Ruth A. Rice

Sherry Richardson

Doug Riley

Karen Rivera

Crystal Roberts

Gary Robertson

Sha Robinson

Cynthia Robison

Suzanne Rodger

Christy Rodgers

Elizabeth Rose

Louann Rose

Mable Ross

Claudia Rossi

Randy Rossiter

Eric Roughtvedt

Rashel Saak

Patricia Sain-Seldin

Ashley Salazar

Nico Salomon

Sherry Salveson

Nalene R. Sanchez

Wanda Sanchez

Susan Sanders

Michelle Santuomo

Kathleen Sayers

Richard Scearcy

Robert Schindler

Hendrik Schroeder

Michael Schultz

Alaine Schumann

Kim Schwindt

Angela Scott

Joyce Scott

Jeanne B. Seaman

JoAnna Secor

Raj Seth

Rainey Shafer

Debbie Shaffer

Erin F. Shaffett

Hallah Shepard

Sherri

Karen L. Shriver

Zaid Siddiqui

Pamela M. Singer

Mary Sjoberg

Dede Smith

Cyndy S. Smith

Jerry Smith

Aminah Smith

David E. Smith

Jenny Smith

Edward Smith

Leona Smith

H. Michael Smith, Jr.

A. C. Smithwick

Jami Snider

Suzan Snook

Stephen Snyder

Darlene M. Snyderr

Robin Sonntag

Lori Soto

Laura Spain

Amy Speed

Erin McBride Spivey

Robert Spivey

Sue Springer

Martha Springsted

If you'd like to join me in the fight, please go to **www.patreon.com/kendberrymd.**

Your help is so important.

CONTENTS

FOREWORD

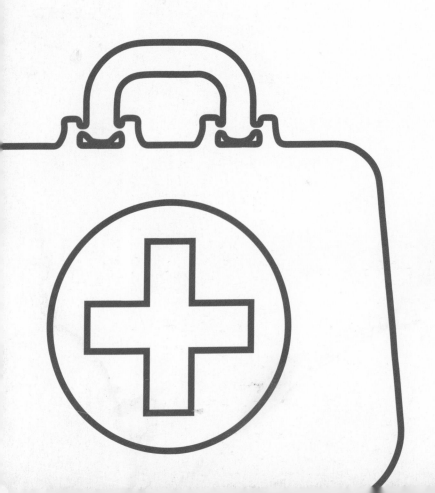

The first time I picked up *Lies My Doctor Told Me*, I immediately recognized someone who had the same fire in his belly as I do. Dr Ken Berry has put down in simple language the tragic idiosyncrasies of medicine that are doing patients harm. That the medical profession continues to perpetuate the spread of certain information is ample justification for the confronting title of *Lies My Doctor Told Me*. It immediately makes you pay attention, and I am fine for that.

_____

Lies My Doctor Told Me is a survival kit for both patients and doctors alike.

This is not a book about "doctor bashing" as much as a resource for all parties to create an open discussion regarding healthy options. Patients want and need to be better informed, and doctors need to be able to discuss openly the information that's widely available to patients. The adage of "Trust me; I am a doctor," no longer has the credibility of yesteryear.

Doctors are becoming far more accountable to their patients, and the only way for doctors to "survive" is to read more, in and around medicine. You may be a doctor and be in complete agreement on what you read in this book. You may, on the other hand, find this text disconcerting, but I can assure you that too many doctors across the globe practice the myths covered in *Lies My Doctor Told Me*. My travels and communications assure me of that.

Patients need to be informed of the misconceptions that lurk out there—particularly in the doctor's office.

The intent of this book is not necessarily to blame individual doctors; rather the purpose is to consider the health-washing of their medical education that has been tainted by vested interests—including the pharmaceutical and food industries—and ideological bias. The more you look, the more you find the agendas of industry and ideology that have affected research outcomes. There is no greater manipulation than in the field of "nutrition science," and *Lies My Doctor Told Me* spends some time denouncing myths in that arena.

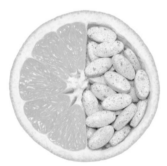

We as a profession are largely to blame. We became confused in believing that "nutrition science" was the same as "medical science." The former has been promoted by the food industry for 100 years and is based around improving profit, palatability, shelf-life, transportability, and, lastly, health. Medical science should be based on the scientific method that incorporates observation, hypothesis, testing, conclusion, and cautious implementation with ongoing review. This remarkable oversight that resulted in linking the two and calling "nutrition science" a "science" may be the biggest human health tragedy of all time.

My journey into the myths of medicine has been like that of Ken's. I had numerous health issues of my own despite following conventional, traditional, and "mythical" guidelines, and I paid the price for that. It was when I started challenging those entrenched dogmas, particularly around nutrition, that I found that virtually everything was a house of cards, collapsing with the simplest of questions of the so-called research and nutrition science.

I am fairly certain that Ken asked me to write this foreword to the updated version of *Lies My Doctor Told Me* for being a fellow doctor who dared to challenge peer-reviewed nutritional guidelines and was "reprimanded" accordingly, with the threat of medical deregistration. I raised the issue of the quality of hospital food and its effect on patient safety, and I was punished accordingly. I was effectively "silenced" from recommending for my patients a diet based on fresh, local, and seasonal produce—essentially meat and vegetables without added sugar, loads of carbohydrates, and nutrient-deficient processed food.

Vested interests working against me included a medical system stuck in its own timeless dogma, a cereal food industry that identified me as a problem, and a medical registration and censorship system that could not bring itself to admit its failings.

With the support of many people in our local and international community, combined with the double-edged sword of social media, common sense finally prevailed. After nearly five years, the determination against me was overturned with a formal apology.

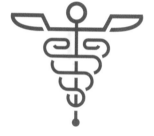

Through social media platforms, Ken and I have become friends, although we've never met directly. We are kindred spirits, and it has been a joy to link with him and other forward-thinking health professionals across our planet. The Internet has closed distances for us all; when we do meet up, there will be plenty of time made to chew the fat.

Lies My Doctor Told Me is something I would have loved to write. I agree with the entire concept. This second edition adds chapters that enhance the wealth of information of the first edition.

Calling out the lies and the perpetrators in any situation is an uncomfortable experience for all, but it's the only way forward in seeking reform. The health, and ultimately the wealth, of modern society is on the line. The future for our children hangs in the balance. I used to be concerned primarily by environmental effects for the future, but that "future" is distant. Our health is in the balance today.

Unfortunately, we are confronted by a health system that does not encourage the lengthy medical consultations that we need for true health education for patients. The business model that accompanies health provision that exists in many countries is just not designed for that "luxury." It suffers from a "medicate or operate" model that has been around for 100 years.

"Half of what you are taught as medical students will in ten years have been shown to be wrong. And the trouble is, none of your teachers know which half." Dr. Sydney Burwell announced this now famous quote at a dinner while he was Dean of Harvard Medical School in the late 1930s. It was provocative then but has endured to this day.

In my thirty-five years as a medical practitioner, at least half of what I can remember from medical school is now defunct. If we continue to accept this concept of knowledge obsolescence, then at least half of our current guidelines are going to be proven incorrect, and therefore potentially harmful to the community.

My concern is that current opinion has become entrenched as guidelines that have become rulebooks for doctors. Dissenters do not get invited to be on guideline-recommendation committees. Challenging those guidelines, which often are influenced by vested pharmaceutical and food industry interests, has become a roadblock to progress.

Many doctors fear the wrath of their governing bodies for taking up the cause for quality assurance, the process of reviewing current practice given current information.

Medicine is at a crossroads, and this time it is about challenging paradigms. Our patients are challenging them for us via the learning fields of social media and the Internet, whether doctors like it or not.

Doctors must be accountable to our patients. You, as a doctor, may not agree with Ken's stand on the issues covered in *Lies My Doctor Told Me*, but you should be aware that the issues are all topical in 2019. Not being able to discuss them with your patients is going to cost you your patients' confidence. I hear from patients almost daily that they don't trust their doctors. That's a far cry from my early days as a consultant.

I am one of those doctors who took the path of resistance against entrenched paradigms, yet that direction was the right path for my patients. Ken reminds us that taking on the "guidelines" can be awkward, but he and I will continue to live and practice by this adage: Science evolves by being challenged. Not by being followed. You are welcome to join us.

Gary Fettke
M.B., B.S., F.R.A.C.S. (Ortho), F.A.Orth.A.
Orthopaedic Surgeon and Low Carbohydrate Healthy Fat (LCHF)
    advocate
Tasmania, Australia

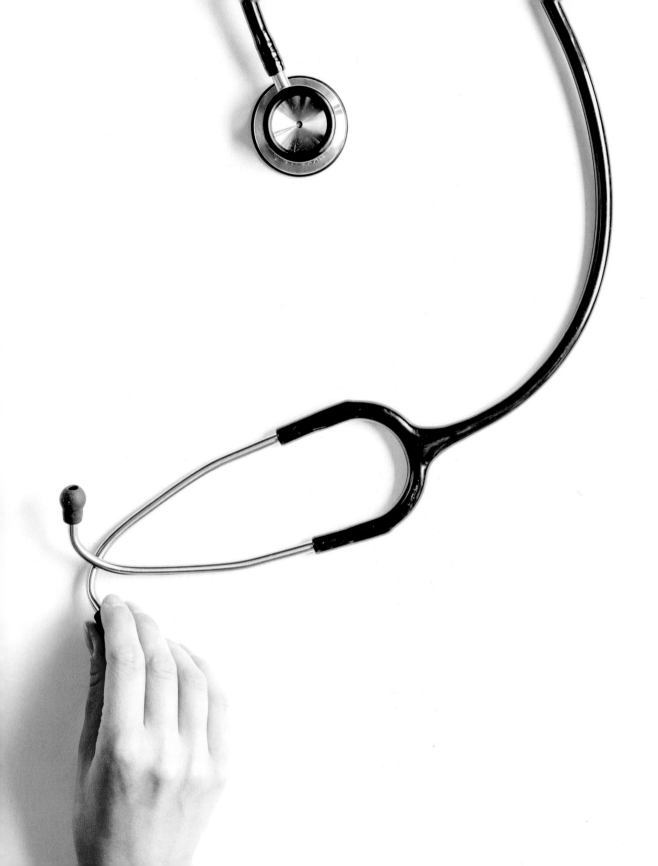

PREFACE

"

The doctor is more to be feared than the disease.

—French proverb

"

This book will upset many doctors; it might even upset *your* doctor. If it does upset your doctor, that's a good sign that either you need to work on the relationship between you and your doctor, or you need to find a new one.

You see, there are two basic types of doctors. The most common type is comfortable where he is. He might read a little to keep up his CME (continuing medical education), but he has no real interest in reading deeply and broadly about medicine. This doctor readily accepts any new guidelines published by medical societies or the federal government. He doesn't care who paid for the research used to "prove" that a new pill works. He only wants to practice medicine with as little effort as possible. He considers himself the boss in the doctor-patient relationship. He believes he holds all the knowledge that matters, and the patient should listen respectfully and not question him.

> **There is often so much politics in medicine that being right can actually get you into trouble.**

If a patient suggests to this kind of doctor that they try something new or consider a new treatment, the doctor will become flustered, impatient, or angry. He doesn't seem to be interested in the uniqueness of each patient. This type of doctor believes he learned all he needed to know in his training and is not interested in continuing to learn. He will belittle, or berate, a patient who suggests that there may be another way to treat something. He is not happy at all if a patient brings information printed from the Internet to discuss with him. He will quickly let the patient know that he is the doctor and doesn't have time for such silliness. This kind of doctor will not like this book at all.

The other type of doctor is an eager learner and a lifelong student. He reads deep in his own specialty, but he also reads about other specialties. He is always considering new treatments as well as ancient ones. This type of doctor is impressed when patients are concerned enough to learn about their symptoms and bring what they find to their office visits. He feels he is the patient's learned partner in health care rather than a dictator. This type of doctor is not offended when a patient speaks of chiropractic, naturopathy, or essential oils. When a patient shares printed information with him, covered in handwritten notes, he is excited because he knows this patient is very interested in their health. This type of doctor will most likely applaud this book.

THIS BOOK IS NOT MEDICAL ADVICE

This book is meant to stimulate thought in both doctors and patients. I want you as a patient to reexamine your health and any medical conditions you have. Are you doing the best you can to optimize your health? Is the advice you've received from doctors the best possible advice? I want you to read, research, and think about your health. Stimulating such action is what this book is for. This book is not medical advice. You should not start, stop, or change any medication based on what you read in this book. You should discuss those types of changes with your trusted doctor. If you don't trust your current doctor, then find a new one.

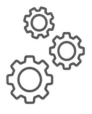

When writing about health and medicine, especially as a doctor, one has to be careful not to give medical advice. This medico-legal term, *medical advice*, refers to information you should receive only in a doctor-patient relationship, not from a book or website. Medical advice is something that can be given only by a provider to a patient in a particular scenario. This advice is given to the patient either in the hospital, clinic, urgent care, or, increasingly, during an online consultation. You should use the information in this book to become an expert on your health and medical conditions. You should use this book to form intelligent questions and requests for your doctor. You should not, however, change your medical regimen based solely on the contents of this book.

HOW TO USE THIS BOOK

You may not want to read this book from cover to cover, and there's no issue if you want to skip around or read only the chapters that apply to your health. Please underline, highlight, and write in this book. Fold down corners and copy and share this book all you want. I want it to help as many people as possible to experience their best health. The end of each chapter includes a homework section. If a chapter doesn't apply to you, then feel free to ignore the homework. If, however, a chapter seems important to your unique health, then the homework section is where you can continue learning about the subject.

WHERE ARE THE WORKS CITED?

The ultimate purpose of this book is to encourage you to do your own thinking. I want you to think about your health and any diagnoses you've been given. To take charge of your health, you need to learn how to research health topics on your own. Because of this, and to keep the size of this book under control, I have omitted footnotes or lists of works cited. I'm not selling anything, so I have no motive to mislead you. I won't be pushing any supplements, powders, or pills on you; I just want you to be awake and aware of your health and the health care offered to you. You can use Bing.com, DuckDuckGo.com, or Google.com to search any health topic.

When you're ready to dive deeper into the medical research, you can go to PubMed.gov, type in your keywords, and search every medical research article in the world. This is the website doctors should use when looking for the latest research on a topic. With your Internet connection, a cup of coffee, and a few hours of research, you can be as knowledgeable as any doctor about your particular health issues. If you can answer your own medical question, then good; if you can't, then print out what you have researched, attach your notes, and take your research to a trusted doctor. He should be happy to discuss with you the information you've found.

PRONOUN USAGE

I debated how I would handle pronouns in this book. English is behind other languages in this area. We often must resort to the awkward *he or she* and *his or her* (as in "He or she should always respect his or her patient"). This is distracting to write and painful to read. Years ago, I had the idea of using *E*. Much as we use capital *I* to talk about ourselves, I thought there should be a way to say "he or she" more easily by using a gender-neutral capital *E*. It would save time and ink and be easier to read (for example, "E should always be respectful of patients"). I had full intention of using E in this book, but decided perhaps people were not ready for that yet. My wife, Neisha, suggested that I pick a pronoun and use it throughout the entire book. We discussed which pronoun I should use and decided a coin-flip would be a fair way to decide. He/his won the toss, and so in this book I use he/his where pronouns are necessary. I will use she/her in the next book.

USE OF THE WORD *DOCTOR*

To make this book easier to read, I use the word *doctor* to refer to all health-care providers. The word *doctor*, as used in this book, can be used interchangeably with nurse practitioner, physician assistant, and nurse-midwife. Any of these health-care providers can tell you medical lies but also are capable of taking your health to the next level by telling you helpful medical truths. Regardless of which kind of provider you see, this book can help you improve your relationship with your health-care provider.

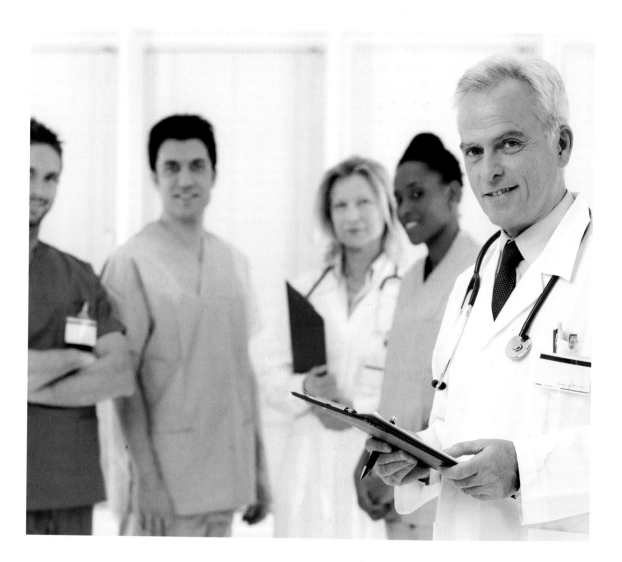

Chapter 1

TRUST IN GOD, NOT YOUR DOCTOR

> # "
> ## Though the doctors treated him, let his blood and gave him medications to drink, he nevertheless recovered.
>
> —Leo Tolstoy, *War and Peace*
>
> "

Do you have a good working relationship with your doctor? If not, you should keep reading. If you do, you still should keep reading because what you are about to learn might strengthen that relationship.

I'm sure your doctor is a caring, kind, and thoughtful individual. However, he isn't superhuman, and he isn't God. Your doctor, at some point, had to possess intelligence and curiosity, or he would not be your doctor today. The path through college, medical school, residency, and medical practice is a very demanding, tricky road. As a result, not everyone can travel it. At some earlier point in his life, your doctor was an energetic, eager-to-learn, ready-to-try-new-things student who couldn't wait to learn everything possible and apply it to improving the health of his patients. What has happened to him since then? How did your doctor go from being an eager, curious learner, to a stuck-in-a-rut, bored, burned-out individual who just spent a whopping three minutes with you for your medical visit? That is a complicated question, and it varies from doctor to doctor.

In the following pages, I attempt to explain the thinking and motivation of your doctor to help you understand what's happening during the average office visit and give you a peek at what's going on behind the scenes and inside the head of your doctor. Let me begin by telling you the story of one doctor I know: me.

I went through medical school with 175 other individuals of all shapes, sizes, ethnicities, and genders. We had all done the work and suffered the hardships to get there for one reason: to become doctors. Some of my friends in medical school were there only because their families had demanded they go to either medical school or law school. Some were there only because they wanted to be the first person in the family to become a doctor. A few of my colleagues in medical school were just there for the money and the prestige. Honestly, those people were few and far between. Most of us had jumped through all the hoops required to get into medical school because we wanted to be important in our patient's lives, do great things, and help lots of people. We wanted to make the world a healthier place.

I, like several of my classmates, was married and had a family as I went through medical school, which made the process much harder than it would have been had I been single. I'm not saying a single person would not have had responsibilities aside from school, but single people would have been less likely to have responsibilities that would have felt slighted or betrayed if

> **"**
> You can lead a doctor to knowledge, but you can't make him think.

the promises made about life on the other side of medical school had not been kept. Medical school requires many hours of study, both solitary and in groups. My home away from home for the first two years was a small four-by-eight-foot room on the seventh floor of the library; it contained only a desk, a chair, and a lamp. I spent many of my waking hours as a young adult sitting and studying in that drab, depressing little study room.

As medical students, we would always vie for the best of these study rooms—the ones with a slightly bigger desk or a newer lamp. A fellow student and I once almost came to blows when I caught him stealing the comfy chair from my study room. It was a chair I had stolen fairly and squarely from another student's study room some months before. Those hours spent in my study room were hours I didn't get to spend with my family. I tried to make all those hours count so that when I became a doctor, I could somehow repay my family for the lost time. My children were growing up every day, and I was missing milestones of their development much more often than I would have liked. However, I had this calling and compulsion to become a doctor and be everything I imagined being a doctor must mean.

The problem with medical students (past and present) is that, unless one of their parents was a doctor, they don't really understand what it means to be a doctor. We had all watched the TV shows and read the books and dreamed the dreams. However, we had no idea what our daily lives would be like when we finished this journey. Looking back now, it seems a little crazy to have worked so hard and so long to attain a career about which we had little understanding of the daily workings.

The day-to-day life of a doctor was a mystery to us, but we still wanted to live it. Many doctors, when they finish this journey, are disheartened and disenchanted with the realities of their new careers. They regret their decision and the years they spent (wasted) making it their reality. However, there are school loans to pay and obligations to meet. The family waiting at home would be confused, dismayed, and disappointed if the new doctor in the family told them that despite the sacrifices they had endured, he wasn't at all happy with this new career. After all the work, sacrifice, and expense to get through medical school, few doctors will walk away from their investment in this career, even if they discover they're miserable living the life of a doctor. You are therefore often left with a disheartened doctor who's doing something he doesn't love and who doesn't have any real interest in doing his best.

Regardless of the reasons why your doctor went to medical school, he is now a doctor—your doctor. You can be sure that his career, no matter how successful it appears to be, is not what he had hoped or dreamed it would be. His daily reality is nothing like the TV shows he watched, the books he read, or the dreams he dreamed. There is too much paperwork to read, millions of words of federal regulations to follow, employees to manage, bills to pay, and likely a family at home begging for more of his time. The weight of such things can stifle even the most brilliant and motivated mind. Instead of looking for the *best way*, a doctor often resorts to accepting the *least bad way* or is forced to comply with the *state-mandated way* of doing things. Primary care doctors are usually too busy to even think of doing any research or considering different or better ways of doing things. Being a doctor, business owner, and parent and doing each job well is more than most mere mortals can manage. Therefore, expecting a doctor to keep up with all the latest research so he can have independent thoughts about his patients' conditions is just too much to ask.

All these pressures and expectations can stifle a person's mind and extinguish any flicker of hope a doctor may have of doing new and great things in medicine. So, what is a poor patient (you) to do? Wake your doctor up. He doesn't voluntarily want to read, study, and think new thoughts. However, if you ask him respectfully, he will probably do it for you. If you word your request properly, you will develop a much stronger relationship with your doctor. You might also improve his partnerships with other patients. Being demanding, pushy, and loud is the opposite of what you should do.

I agree with what you're probably thinking: It shouldn't be your job to coddle and coax your doctor into going the extra mile for you and your health. However, even though your doctor's apathy toward learning new information is not your *fault*, it is your *problem*. You have only one life and one body to live it in, so you have to take ownership of helping your doctor to help you. If you take charge of the care of your body, you could avoid years of suffering and disease. I know, from being in the trenches of medical practice for more than a decade, what works and what doesn't when it comes to converting your doctor back into a curious, eager learner who is willing to work with you.

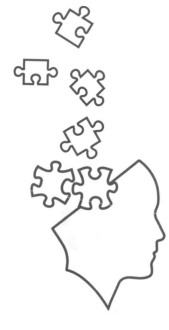

For years, I've had patients try every trick and strategy they could think of to get what they wanted from me, both good things and bad things. If what they wanted was a medication they didn't need, my answer was and still is, "This isn't Burger King; you can't have it your way." If what they wanted was for me to help them take their health and well-being to the next level, then I was more than willing to assist. I'm already receptive to alternative options and the ideas of optimization and true prevention, but most doctors are not. How can you tell whether your doctor is willing to learn? How can you find a doctor who is open to your ideas about your health?

The most powerful and most deceptive medical lie of all is that your doctor knows everything there is to know about your health or about medicine in general. A corollary to this lie is that medical scientists and researchers have discovered everything worth knowing about the human body and human health. As a doctor, I can tell you it would be nice to know everything. It's nice when patients place their trust in me and assume that I know everything. However, as a young doctor, I realized that not only were there many things I didn't know but there also were many things my mentors and professors didn't know. Doctors often carry themselves as if they know everything worth knowing. This is human nature. However, as a patient, you cannot let yourself be deluded into believing this. Your doctor is only as good as the knowledge he possesses and the effort he puts into staying current by looking for further knowledge and updates.

It's common for today's doctors to believe they have learned everything worth knowing. As a result, there seems to be little value in continuing the strenuous study they were used to in medical school. This way of thinking is the rule for most doctors in practice. Most of them will admit that they don't know details of new studies coming out, but they feel confident that the bedrock of their knowledge is solid and without cracks. State medical societies and boards aren't proactive about encouraging doctors to remain current in their studies. Also, the societies and boards do too much to prevent doctors from thinking outside the box or trailblazing new treatments or therapies.

Nothing will start a group of doctors grumbling quicker than mentioning that more continuing medical education should probably be required. The grumbling is about more than just not wanting to be told what to do. Many doctors have a real problem with cramming new knowledge into brains they already consider full. Even worse than a patient who believes their doctor knows everything is a doctor who believes this foolishness about himself. These issues are what you will be up against as you try to forge a meaningful partnership with your doctor or try to find one worth partnering with.

You can lead a doctor to knowledge, but you can't make him think. It's rare to find a doctor who stays energized and excited about the field of medicine and caring for patients. Most doctors quickly become comfortable in the rut of their medical practice. As a result, they learn only the bare minimum needed to stay current with their medical society's requirements, and they do even that begrudgingly. Doctors are not bad or evil; they're simply human. To get the most out of this book, you need to realize several things. These things might seem simple-minded and obvious at first, but please think about each one. The main reason this book is necessary is that most patients and doctors have forgotten the following important facts.

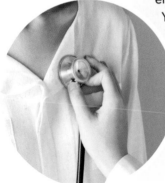

You have only one life.
Your life is not a video game or a movie. Every decision you make about your health or allow your doctor to make for you, whether well-thought-out or foolish, can have an enormous effect on your long-term health and happiness. You don't get extra credit for blindly believing your doctor. You don't get a free pass just because your doctor told you to do something. If your doctor gives you bad advice, and you apply it to your health, it's you and your family who suffer, either a little or a lot, and perhaps for the rest of your life. Even if you can prove the doctor's error in court and successfully sue him for millions, you will still be the one left without some part of your health.

Your doctor is human.

Your doctor, despite his reputation or your belief in him, is only human, just like you. He is motivated by the same things that you are. He has the same weaknesses and makes the same sorts of mistakes. In spite of this truth, you should still hold your doctor to a higher standard. He should study and think harder than most other people you know. He should also strive to remain current on a variety of medical subjects. However, you cannot blindly assume he does this; you must make sure. Only by establishing a partnership and building trust with a doctor will you be able to decipher whether he is an eager, lifelong student or doing the bare minimum to get by.

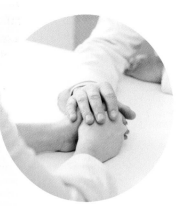

The doctor-patient relationship should be a partnership.

You should expect your doctor to have the latest and best medical knowledge. His job is to sift through tons of medical studies and textbooks and even to read far and wide outside the field of medicine. This research enables him to provide medical advice that is customized just for you—advice that honors your DNA and ensures that you have the best chance for a long, healthy life. You should expect your doctor not to give you incorrect or outdated advice. You should expect your doctor not to offer you a new pill just because of the slick ads and charming drug reps sent to him by Big Pharma. You should never blindly accept your doctor's advice, and you should trust your intuition about your health. You find true health by blending research, your health intuition, and your doctor's learned advice.

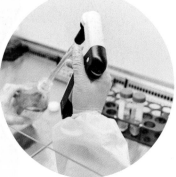

Research studies never tell the whole story.

Your doctor's job is to know this. However, because many doctors do such a poor job at extra study, and because your one life is at stake, you have to help. The Internet puts all the latest research within your reach. Therefore, to use this information to your best advantage, you should have a basic understanding of how medical research is conducted and, perhaps more importantly, who pays for it. Only so much medical research is conducted at any given time. This research costs billions of dollars to conduct, and someone must pay for it. Consequently, most medical research is paid for by Big Government or Big Pharma. Either choice has serious drawbacks. For scientists to conduct meaningful research, their thinking must be impartial and unbiased. Impartial and unbiased thinking is seldom used by Big Government and never used by Big Pharma.

No one can keep up with all the research.

So much medical research is published today that no doctor can possibly keep up with it all. A good doctor sifts through as much of this research as possible and decides which studies give useful conclusions that he can apply to the health of his patients. Conversely, he also must decide which studies are thinly veiled pseudoscience performed by Big Pharma to get their next billion-dollar baby (drug) approved by the FDA. A good doctor looks for and finds meaningful research within his specialty. A great doctor also searches for information from other specialties and other branches of science. This search for information he can use to prevent disease and to optimize your health should be his all-consuming calling.

This book is not an indictment of doctors.

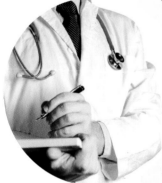

Remember, I am a doctor. I don't intend to make doctors out to be the bad guys. My goal is to call attention to very correctable problems in the current thinking of most doctors and how they are educated. This book should serve as a wake-up call for both doctors and patients. Both groups need to step it up a notch.

Doctors, it is your job to remain as up-to-date as possible on current research and not to believe every word that comes out of Big Pharma–sponsored research or the charismatic drug rep's mouth.

Patients, this is your one life we're talking about. Nothing is more important to your long-term health than your diet and lifestyle. Stop being mentally and physically lazy. Stop blindly trusting your doctor and Big Pharma to give you a magic pill to fix the health problems your diet has caused. Stop expecting your doctor to have a magic treatment to correct the damage your lifestyle is doing. Think about your health, research the latest options, think about solutions, and ask your doctor thoughtful questions. If your doctor becomes upset by all your questions, then your partnership might not be working. It might be time to repair it or to look for a new partner. If you blindly take the advice of your doctor and he is wrong, you and your family will suffer. Doctors who give bad advice have a way, just like everyone else, of placing the blame elsewhere. Most doctors won't lose a minute of sleep if your health suffers because you followed their bad advice.

Your health is both robust and fragile at the same time. If your diet and lifestyle are correct, you almost can't get sick. If your diet and lifestyle are incorrect, you almost can't get well. You're the product of thousands of successful reproductions. Your DNA is the product of an awesome creation and the culmination of many generations of improving stock. All it takes is one wrong prescription or one unneeded medical test, and you could suffer a side effect that will devastate your health or end your life. You should never trust something so precious and valuable as your health to the opinion of one person—not even your doctor.

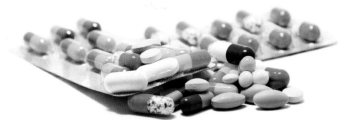

Chapter 2

SO WHAT'S GOING ON HERE?

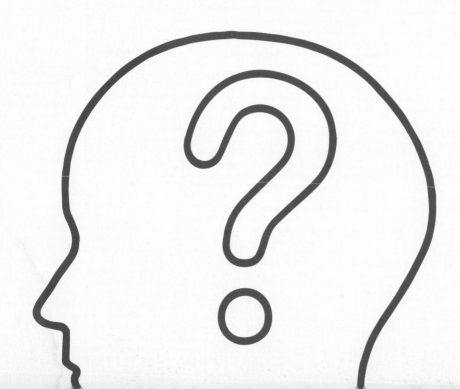

> ## The life so short, the craft so long to learn.
>
> —Hippocrates

Who am I, anyway? I am a board-certified medical doctor, recently accepted as a fellow in the American Academy of Family Medicine, which is kind of a big deal for a family doctor. I've been practicing medicine in a small Southern town for more than a decade and have slowly become more and more aware of the failings of modern medicine. If you break your leg or rupture your appendix, modern medicine is what you need. If you are relatively healthy and are interested in both optimizing your health and working toward true, meaningful prevention of disease, then modern medicine will probably let you down.

I am planted firmly in the middle of both the good and the bad that is modern medicine. I never wanted to be part of the problem, but looking back now, it's obvious I was. The small, rural county in which I have practiced my entire career was recently named one of the unhealthiest counties in Tennessee, which made me feel like a failure. I was getting paid well to set a terrible example and give terrible advice to my patients. When I started my practice, I was young and thin, and I was in superb health. As the years went by, my diet kept getting worse, and I was always too busy to be more active.

A few years into my career, I had my lab values checked and was shocked to find that I was becoming diabetic. That was not something I was okay with at all. One day, I got short of breath trying to tie my shoes. I've always tried to give good advice and set a good example, but it became apparent that I was doing neither. I realized it was both comical and embarrassing that I was telling patients every day that they needed to lose weight while my belly made it look like I might go into labor at any moment.

My "waking up" has been a years-long process, starting with the self-discovery that I was an obese doctor who expected my patients to take my advice about weight loss and health. I started applying my natural inclination and ability to question everything and accept nothing blindly to the study of medicine for the first time. The deeper I researched, the more I realized just how ignorant I was. I've always had the natural ability (some would call it a curse) to question what the experts in any field say. Sometimes this ability gets me into trouble. However, this time it cleared the way for me to become a better doctor. Since our bodies are made of the food we've eaten, I thought nutrition would be a great place to start. I dug through the boxes containing all my notes from medical school, pulled out everything I had been taught about nutrition, and looked it over.

Because nutrition is so important to good health, I'm sure you are imagining a huge stack of books and notes on my desk, right? Instead, I found only one half semester's worth of notes and a small paperback book. I could hold it all comfortably in one hand. No joke—that's the total of what the 175 of us learned about nutrition in four years of medical school. A biochemistry professor who was a native of New Zealand had given most of our nutrition lectures. All I could remember was his accent and the interesting

> "Patients should be able to trust their doctors to be intellectually honest. They aren't paying for good-sounding random answers to their medical questions.

way he said pasta (paasssta). I remember how he said the word both because of the way he said it and because of the number of times he said it.

During his few lectures, he shared with us that he was a brittle diabetic. He also told us about the many servings of whole-wheat pasta he ate daily, trying to keep his blood sugar under control. As a medical student, I did not understand how the two were related or how ridiculous his statement was. The lesson we medical students learned was that somehow lots of servings of whole-wheat pasta must be good for diabetics. Looking in the mirror at my fat belly, I realized that eating lots of whole-wheat pasta wasn't working for my patients or me. Increasingly convinced that I was ignorant of the nutrition needed to nourish the human body, I studied nutrition for the first time in my medical career.

First, I assumed that studying nutrition textbooks and journals would be the proper approach. I quickly realized that big food corporations sponsor publication of most of this information, and the publications offer little that would help in prevention and healing. Next, I looked at the Atkins Diet. In medical school, we learned that this diet could be bad for your kidneys, and we were told we probably shouldn't recommend it to patients. When I looked at the research the first time, the conclusions of most of the studies seemed to support this belief. When I looked again, this time at the whole of the research and not just the conclusions of the studies, I realized that the findings didn't support the conclusions. It was a weird awakening for me as a doctor. It's common practice for a busy doctor to read only the conclusion of a research paper, not the entire paper. Doctors do this because of their justifiable assumption that the conclusion should honestly sum up the research, findings, and take-home message of the research in a few hundred words.

It turns out that the researchers often slant the conclusions of studies toward what the researcher thinks or wants the study to show or not show. Even worse, conclusions are often tainted by the desires of the Big Pharma or Big Food corporation that sponsored the study. I decided the Atkins Diet wasn't as dangerous as I'd been led to believe. Therefore, I tried it myself. I lost 20 pounds in two months, and my kidney function was better than it had been before I started! My problem with the Atkins Diet was that I actually like veggies and berries and missed eating them. I got bored eating rib-eye steak and butter all the time (true story). I looked at the South Beach Diet, the Ornish Diet, and a few others. Then I found a book called *The Primal Blueprint* by Mark Sisson. It spoke to me and changed my paradigm about nutrition, health, and medicine. This diet tried to mimic a primal or Paleo diet, like the one our ancestors ate thousands of years ago.

Here's the thinking that sold me on primal/Paleo as the best possible way for humans to eat and live. Human DNA has been on this planet for thousands of years. It survived and thrived while people commonly ate certain things and never ate other things. If our distant ancestors made it through childbirth and dodged infectious diseases and predators, they seemed to stay healthy and live robustly into old age. Only with the introduction of grains, sugars, and other starches as a large part of our daily diet did we begin to get fat and sick (with chronic noninfectious diseases). I memorized *The Primal Blueprint* and tried to live by it as best I could. I lost another 20 pounds and started having fun and enjoying life again. I didn't feel the need to work out anymore; I would just go outside and play like a kid. I was going through family and social changes, yet they didn't get me down and make me angry like they would have when I was fat. It was almost as if changing my diet had changed my mood, attitude, and outlook as well.

Since then, I have read many more books about human nutrition, including *The Paleo Diet, The Paleo Solution,* and *The Bulletproof Diet.* My diet and lifestyle are a blend of all those concepts. Currently, I'm investigating intermittent fasting, thermogenics, and optimization of my gut bacteria as ways to further improve my health and mood. When I find something that works and is safe, I share it with my patients. So, you see, doctors can wake up and get out of their little boxes if they try. You might even be able to wake up your doctor.

So, what's wrong with your doctor? Let me first reassure you that your doctor is probably a well-meaning, thoughtful, and caring person who wants the best for you. All doctors start out this way. Although these traits get buried and sometimes become dormant, I'm sure they're still in there somewhere. Doctors are very, very busy people. There are pressures and expectations on them that you might not imagine. There are hundreds of pages of medical journals to read weekly and thousands of pages of government/insurance regulation updates to read monthly—not to mention a practice (small business) to run, social expectations to manage, and family to spend time with.

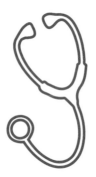

I don't say this to make excuses for your doctor. I say this to remind you that your doctor is human. He has only so much time, effort, and brains to go around. Unfortunately, it's human nature to look for shortcuts when you're overstretched, overstressed, and overpromised. Let me describe for you some of the shortcuts your doctor might be taking that could affect your health. Keep in mind that your doctor takes these shortcuts not because he's mean, dishonest, or part of some conspiracy. He does it because there are only so many hours in a day, and he can't do everything.

THE LAWS OF HUMAN NATURE THAT APPLY TO YOUR DOCTOR

Doctors are human (at least for now), and as such, they are just as liable to fall victim to errors of thinking, of taking shortcuts, and of being, well . . . human as any of the rest of us. This is why my first chapter reminded you to have faith in God but not your doctor. Doctors are on average very smart people, but that doesn't make them infallible or above suspicion. Just ask any state medical board. Medical boards are suspicious of all doctors, especially those who step outside the box or dare to try something new. Here are a few thought-errors your doctor probably falls victim to.

When the only tool you have is a hammer, everything looks like a nail.

This is an important law of human nature. You should understand this idea as it relates to your doctor, your mechanic, and every other expert in your life. Abraham Maslow and others describe this idea as the *law of the instrument*. Maslow noted that if you give a young child a hammer, then the child will hammer everything that's within the child's reach. Let me explain how this applies to your doctor: We all understand what a hammer is and what it does to a nail. However, you should consider that tools not only help us do work but also affect the way we think about the work we do. As a result, the tools we have available can alter how we go about doing our work.

If a carpenter has only a hammer and nails, then he will think about nailing things to whatever he is doing. If all he has is a saw, then he will think about ways of cutting off pieces of what he is working on. This was a great strategy back in the Paleolithic days, when human beings had limited tools. It helped them figure out how to take a stick or a rock (the only tool they might have had) and knock fruit out of a tree, so they didn't starve. Today, however, we have multiple tools at our disposal. Some tools are good, and some are not so good. However, this way of thinking is still hard-wired into our brains. As a result, it can cause us to use the wrong tool. We tend to consider using only the tools we have readily available and the tools we have already learned how to use to get our work done.

Here's an example of how this way of thinking could affect your doctor: A family doctor advising an obese diabetic would probably say that the patient needs to cut back on calories, eat less fat and more whole grains, and exercise more. The doctor might also prescribe a daily pill or three to take. The *tools* this doctor has easy access to are the nutrition *facts* he learned in medical school and his prescription pad. He's too busy to learn about other tools that he could use to help this patient. Therefore, the patient gets the benefit of only the tools his doctor knows about and chooses to use. A surgeon advising that same obese diabetic might say that the patient needs stomach-bypass surgery to cure his diabetes and obesity. The tool of a surgeon is surgery, so that is what the surgeon tells the patient he needs. An endocrinologist (a doctor who specializes in glands and diabetes) who sees the same patient would probably give the patient an insulin pump and a prescription for some of the most expensive medications on the market. Those are the tools that this expert uses daily, and thus the ones he is proficient at using. All three scenarios involve the same patient, but each expert uses a different *tool* to help the patient. You should be saying, "I wonder if other tools exist that would work better for this patient that weren't used at all."

Good thought! Each doctor is using the tools he's comfortable with. These doctors are neither considering each patient as a unique individual nor are they looking for new (or old) tools that might work better than their current tools. How should we feel about these three doctors? Should we judge them, hate them, praise them, or ignore them? These behaviors don't make the family doctor, the surgeon, or the endocrinologist bad or dishonest. They just make them human. There are other tools available to help this patient, but these doctors use only the tools they currently know about and believe in. Only a doctor who is constantly reading and learning, and who often does research outside of his specialty or even outside the field of medicine, will discover better tools.

Learning about new tools is time-consuming and full of dead ends. You may invest hours studying some new tool only to find that it doesn't work, is too expensive, or is just too dangerous to use. Doctors learn to be stingy with their time, and rightfully so. They have only so much time, and some portion of it is already spoken for. Also, as the saying goes, time is money. Time a doctor spends searching for a better tool means less time to use his existing tools to make money. Therefore, you can understand why a doctor might choose not to look for new tools or might ignore a new tool that is unproven or not approved by his medical board, his professional society, or the FDA.

When your income depends on believing a certain thing, you tend to believe it.

Upton Sinclair once wrote, "It is difficult to get a man to understand something when his salary depends upon his not understanding it." This law of human nature sounds dishonest on its face. However, it doesn't necessarily mean that your doctor is dishonest. The way the current system is set up, a family doctor will never get in trouble with the state medical board for telling you to eat fewer calories, eat whole grains, eat low-fat, and eat less salt—even though this counseling has been shown in multiple meaningful studies to be terrible advice and to almost never work. His income and his future as a doctor are perfectly safe if he repeats this foolishness daily for the rest of his career. This advice helps no one. All his patients end up feeling guilty and give up because it's impossible for them to follow this advice. The surgeon will never get into trouble with the state medical board for performing bariatric surgery, even though his patients can end up with long-term problems and very uncomfortable lives. They can even gain back the weight, assuming they have no devastating surgical complications in the operating room (a signed waiver legally protects the surgeon from these). The endocrinologist is safe with the medical board when he prescribes an insulin pump, even in a patient whose pancreas still makes insulin. He is even safe in prescribing medications so expensive that the patient is guaranteed never to be able to afford them.

Now, let's suppose that a doctor, through thinking, reading, and researching, comes up with a diet plan, pill, or shot that will cure this overweight diabetic patient permanently. What can, and what should, he do with this treatment?

If this good doctor started trying to tell the world about this new tool to cure obesity and diabetes, how would he go about it? In our culture, he would advertise. That is how we spread the word about new discoveries from which other people could benefit. Therefore, this doctor would take out ads in the newspaper, get a website, create a Facebook page, and proceed to tell the world about this new tool he has discovered. He would proudly proclaim to the world that none of the other tools doctors had told them about were necessary. They need only use his new tool, and their obesity and diabetes would go away so they could be healthy and happy. Can you guess what would happen next? This doctor would quickly receive a not-so-nice letter from his medical board telling him to stop advertising his tool immediately. Even worse, he might even receive a summons from the board with the threat of a fine. The medical board might even take action against his medical license—such as suspending or revoking it—even if his tool does, in fact, work better than every other tool out there. Regardless of whether it's the best tool ever invented to cure obesity and diabetes, the medical board wouldn't care or want to hear about it. I'm telling you a true story, my friends.

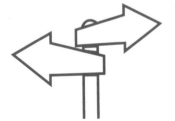

Humans (doctors) are always looking for shortcuts in every part of their lives.

We all love shortcuts, and that's one reason we live in a modern society in which we have a machine to do almost every task for us. As discussed previously, one seemingly useful time-saving shortcut that doctors take is to read only the conclusions in the many medical journals they skim; they don't read entire articles. The reason is that most medical studies, when published, are broken into parts, including the abstract, background, methods, and conclusion. Summarizing only the conclusion is also what the news media does when it reports on medical studies with the intent to scare you. Often, when I hear a news report on one of these studies, I have to roll my eyes. It's obvious that someone with no medical training has read only the conclusion or someone else's summary of the conclusion. The conclusions of medical research studies often don't truly represent what the study's results revealed.

Another shortcut that doctors take is to lump patients into several groups. Then, when they encounter an individual patient who seems to fit into one of these groups, the answer to the question of which prescription pill to give is obvious. For this type of doctor, there is no such thing as a unique patient; there are just different types of patients. Thinking is hard work, and if a doctor is a little lazy or a lot overstretched, this shortcut seems well worth it in the short term. Obviously, though, with these shortcuts, the patient is often shortchanged and can even be harmed.

Association seems to imply causation.

Just because there's an association between two things does not mean that one of those things causes the other thing to happen. This concept is hard to understand and to keep in mind. Sometimes it seems that because two things are related, one thing must have caused the other thing. For example, your parents might have told you to stay away from the bad kids because they believed that good kids who hung out with bad kids would become bad kids themselves.

A medical example of this philosophy is the story of HDL cholesterol. Medical studies have shown that having a high HDL ("good") cholesterol level is associated with a lower risk of heart attack. Therefore, it would seem like a good idea to give patients a pill to raise their HDL level. That should decrease their risk of having a heart attack, right? Doctors have tried this, but the subsequent research found that giving someone a pill to raise their HDL level did not lower their risk of heart attack. High HDL and low heart attack rates are related, but raising a person's HDL does not lower his heart attack risk. High HDL levels are associated with a reduced heart attack risk, but they do not *cause* the decreased risk.

Another example is when a parent brings a sick child with a runny nose and a cough to the doctor. He prescribes the child a course of antibiotics, and a few days later, the child is feeling much better. It appears to the parent that the antibiotics cured the child's illness. In fact, the viral infection causing the illness would have improved in the same amount of time without the antibiotics. Even though the antibiotics seemed associated with the cure, they did not cause the cure.

There once was a study showing that swimming pool drownings were associated with the number of Nicholas Cage movies released during that same time. Even though there was an association between these two things, you would have to be a little unstable to think the drownings were Mr. Cage's fault. The numbers were just a coincidence. In this example, it's easy to see that the two variables (drownings and Cage movies) can't possibly be related. However, in medicine, it's sometimes much harder to tell (HDL levels and heart attack rates).

I would love it if every person on the planet understood this error in thinking, but I don't expect that to happen. I do expect every doctor in medical practice to understand this concept completely and never to be fooled by it. That's a reasonable expectation because most doctors learn about this error in thinking early in their training. However, I'd say that they're not taught well enough; it's one of the most common errors I see doctors make. Still, I do expect every doctor to see through Big Pharma's advertising, which sometimes craftily exploits this error, and not subject their patients to unnecessary pills because of those misleading ads.

When something *sounds* true, we often start believing that it *is* true.

We've all heard the story about George Washington chopping down the cherry tree, but it's an historical lie. Sometimes, when a lie sounds like it should be true and people repeat it often enough, even experts in the field begin to believe the lie and repeat it. Even doctors do this. Just as many teachers through the decades have *taught* their students the lie about George and his naughty hatchet, doctors sometimes *teach* their patients medical lies that are harmful. When we learn a medical lie from a doctor, it can affect our health in negative ways.

Medical lies don't usually start this way, but it is how a few of them have been born. The problem is that when an expert tells a medical lie—whether it's your doctor, the ADA, the FDA, the AMA, or the USDA—patients tend to believe it blindly. The patients then repeat it and keep repeating it for years, even after the experts have disproved it and stop repeating it themselves. Experts very seldom (and by "seldom" I mean *never*) retract their previous opinions in a meaningful public way when they've been proven wrong by further research. The experts just stop repeating the lie and move on with their careers as if nothing had happened. You, as a patient, would have no way of discovering this change in expert opinion without doing hours of research on your own. Therefore, you continue to believe the lie. This is what I call the *echo of the lie*.

A lie keeps echoing through society even after it has been proven false.

When researchers realize that what they'd been publishing as truth in their studies is false, they don't issue a press release to apologize and ask everyone to forgive them for the error. They just stop repeating the lie and move on to the next thing. It's a huge nonevent. They don't want to admit publicly that they were wrong, and no one makes them, so they don't. For example, where are all the doctors pleading for forgiveness on bended knee because they told us for years that we shouldn't eat butter? They're nowhere to be found. They've already moved on to other medical topics while leaving the rest of us confused about what happened. You'll never read a published retraction, a public apology, or even a good explanation about where they went wrong, and you'll never receive a promise that they'll never do it again.

They just moved on, which is understandable because no one wants to admit they were wrong. However, because the perpetrators of the lie are experts, they're causing harm by not correcting the lie. The lie continues to echo through society, sometimes for decades, continuing to harm or inconvenience patients. For example, even after researchers quietly backed away from the eggs-are-bad-for-you lie, it kept being repeated by the media and doctors for years. When the scientists and most of the media (but not all) had stopped telling this lie, it was still repeated by primary care doctors, spouses, parents, and know-it-all neighbors for many more years. To this day, I still have the occasional patient who will argue with me that eggs are full of cholesterol and bad, so they shouldn't eat them. When I tell them to stop eating cereal and milk for breakfast and to eat eggs instead, they look confused and mutter, "But I thought eggs were bad?" This question makes me want to climb a few ivory towers and slap some experts (figuratively, of course). The researchers should have made as big a deal, and just as big a press release, of revealing to the world that their original conclusions about eggs were wrong as they did when they made the original incorrect announcement. If the experts were searching for truth rather than recognition, they would have willingly advertised the change in opinion.

If something is less bad, then it must be good.

Two arguments I deal with in more detail later in this book are that whole wheat is better for you than processed wheat, and raw milk is better for you than processed milk in a carton. When I present the research on these two arguments, you will see that, in fact, whole-wheat foods are less bad for you than processed-wheat foods. In the same way, raw milk (properly collected and stored) is less bad for you than processed milk. However, just because something is less bad for you does not mean that it's good for you. Less bad *does not* equal good. This is an error in thinking that doctors make all the time.

If we did a medical study comparing the health effects of smoking unfiltered cigarettes versus smoking filtered cigarettes, what do you think we would find? Of course, filtered cigarettes (assuming the filter is made of something safe) should cause less disease than unfiltered cigarettes. You, as the researcher, would publish your results in a medical journal with a title such as "Filtered Cigarette Usage Leads to 15.3% Fewer Lung Cancers," and you would feel like you had made the world a better place. A news outlet or government agency publishes a story about your interesting little article, and their story is titled "Filtered Cigarettes Are Much Healthier than Unfiltered." Finally, the local news stations, smaller websites, and parents everywhere tell the world, "Filtered cigarettes are good for you!" Do you see what happened there? In your research, you never meant to claim that filtered cigarettes were actually *good* for people. You were just studying two variables and reporting your findings. Sadly, once your findings had filtered down through doctors, the government, and the media, they had been turned into a lie. This sort of transformation happens all the time in medical research, and it's your doctor's job to detect it and protect you from it.

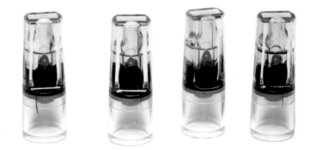

Mindless repetition of a lie makes people believe it.

When your neighbor, Bob, tells you something like, "Trust me; the more you exercise, the more weight you will lose," he's not breaking any rules. Regular people get to say whatever they want, whether they know what they're talking about or not. You can't hold Bob liable for this error, and you can't sue him for damages. He was just stating his opinion on the matter. If your hairdresser tells you, "Honey, you shouldn't eat seeds and popcorn; it will flare up your diverticulitis!" then it is up to you to decide how much she learned about the human colon in her cosmetology classes. She isn't an expert in the medical field, and she doesn't have to be right, or even try to be right, when she shares information. Both Bob and your hairdresser are repeating things they've heard, things that sound correct to them, so they then pass these little nuggets along to you and everyone else who will listen.

For regular folks, this behavior is perfectly acceptable. You shouldn't be surprised if they're often wrong. Doctors, however, should be held to a higher standard. They should either be certain that they know the right information or realize that they might not know and tell you as much. When doctors repeat medical lies, people do get hurt, and the doctor can be held responsible.

When your doctor mindlessly repeats something he read in a medical journal or something he was taught in medical school twenty-five years ago without thinking about you as a unique patient, he's doing you a great disservice. He should be held accountable for his lack of effort. He is neither your neighbor nor is he your chatty hairdresser; he's a licensed expert in human health who's tasked with the responsibility of giving you the best medical advice available. You have every right to expect that your doctor knows what he's talking about when he speaks. Your doctor, as a licensed expert, doesn't have the lazy luxury of repeating something without knowing if it's true. He has a sworn duty to read the medical journals and the relevant studies (in their entirety, not just the conclusions), and even to read outside the field of medicine. Doing so will help him see the bigger picture concerning the health and well-being of his patients. It will also keep him from mindlessly repeating the latest guidelines from Big Government or Big Pharma without stopping to think whether they are based in meaningful research.

When doctors fail us in this most basic area of trust, they also lose credibility in other areas. A doctor should willingly tell his patient when he doesn't know something if that is the case, and he should say that he'll research the issue and report back when he does know. Patients should be able to trust their doctors to be intellectually honest. They aren't paying for good-sounding random answers to their medical questions. They deserve well-thought-out, researched answers that apply to their unique cases. This tendency to perpetuate medical lies is the reason, above all others, I wrote this book. Patients deserve a doctor who will either know the answer, find out the answer, or refer them to a specialist. A patient never deserves a thoughtless canned answer that might or might not be true. A doctor should never repeat a medical lie he has heard or read to his patient, call it medical advice, and be held blameless for it. Those days are over.

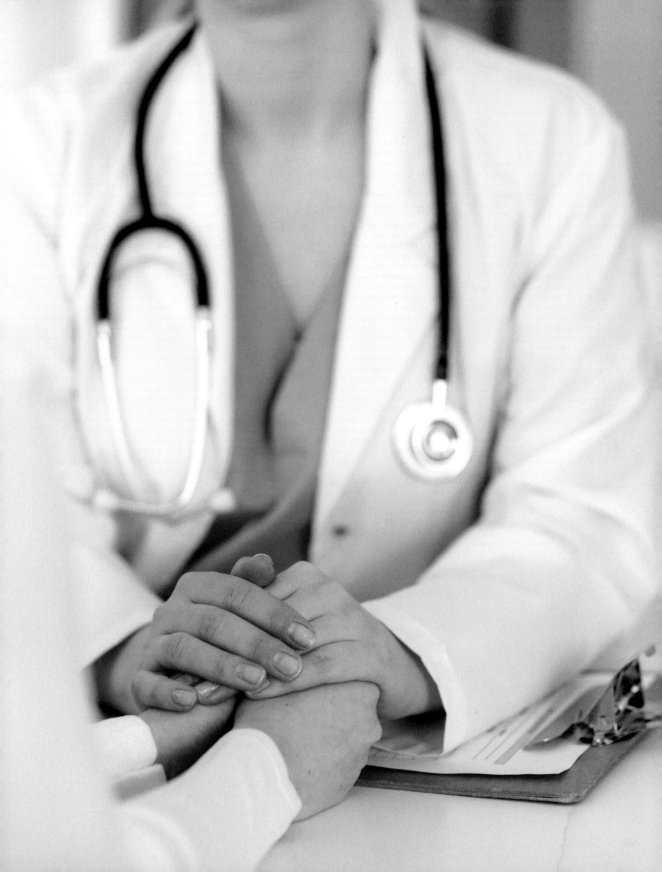

Chapter 3
THE SKINNY ON FAT

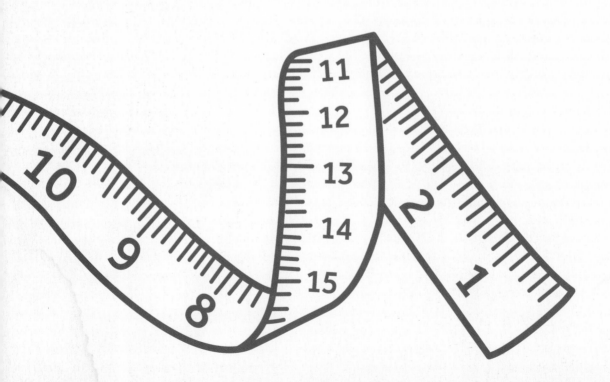

" Unless we put medical freedom in the Constitution, the time will come when medicine will organize itself into an undercover dictatorship. To restrict the art of healing to doctors and deny equal privileges to others will constitute the Bastille of medical science. All such laws are UN-American and despotic.

—Benjamin Rush

THE LIE

Eating fat, especially saturated fat, leads to high cholesterol, obesity, and heart disease.

WHY YOU SHOULD CARE

If fat in our diet does lead to high cholesterol, obesity, and heart disease, then we should avoid it at all costs. If, however, this tasty food has been falsely accused, then wouldn't you like to enjoy it at your liberty? If it's good for you, then wouldn't you want to eat more fat, not less? This important question in the fields of nutrition and medicine needs to be answered with meaningful research and common sense.

SUPPORT FOR THE LIE

All experts, federal government agencies, and academies eagerly repeat this medical lie. It seems so self-evident to the well-meaning experts that dietary fat equals body fat that there is little need for actual thought or research on this subject. If you look for the actual hard research, however, you'll find very little support for this lie. Multiple large studies over the years, which were conducted to show once and for all that eating fat was bad for you, have repeatedly shown no link between fat consumption and increased risk of heart attack or stroke.

THE COMMON SENSE

In few areas of human health and nutrition have medical scientists been more completely and embarrassingly derelict than on the topic of fat nutrition. Something as basic as what human beings should eat to be healthy is still a mystery in the twenty-first century. Or is it? Experts would have us believe that we need to fill up on whole grains and wash them down with glasses of skim milk and fruit juice. These same experts tell us that we should turn away from all saturated fats. However, the evidence for this advice is lacking.

Common sense is defined by Webster.com as "sound and prudent judgment based on a simple perception of the situation or facts." What sense could be more common than thinking we should follow the same diet and behavior that our ancestors followed for thousands of years? These hardy ancestors of ours were hunter-gatherers and didn't stay in one place long enough to grow and genetically modify grains or grasses. They moved around and ate what they could get their hands on. They probably wouldn't have touched skim milk, had it been a choice. They went out of their way to eat fat, breaking open bones for marrow and skulls for brains.

The DNA you carry in every cell of your body was formed and perfected in the harsh environment that was your ancestors' lives. For thousands of years, that DNA was tweaked and perfected on certain foods, green things, protein, and fat, but it never encountered other foods (grains, fruit juice, and skim milk). Therefore, the true commonsense thinking on this topic would be to honor your DNA and eat as much like your ancestors as is practical and possible. Unfortunately, most of us don't do this because the experts stepped in a few decades ago and lied to us.

A *pseudo-commonsense* idea has hijacked this topic: Because the fat in foods and the adipose tissue on our bodies are called by the same word (fat), most people (and most doctors) childishly assume they are the same. As a result, the assumption is that eating one fat, in your food, must lead directly to the production of the other fat, in your body. Although this logic might satisfy a yearning for symmetry and simple arithmetic in the mind of the average person, we should justifiably expect a much higher standard from our nutrition experts and doctors. It's neither their lot nor their privilege to accept anything blindly as fact without rigorous study and trial, even if it sounds like perfect common sense. The job of doctors is to think and to study and to prove or disprove what they and everyone else thinks they know to be true.

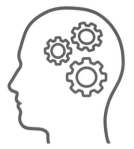

With regard to this medical lie, and several others, doctors have let their patients down and embarrassed themselves by continuing to claim that they're experts on the subject. Many a patient has been deprived of the taste and nourishment of the fats our ancestors enjoyed because a well-intentioned doctor or dietitian said it was bad for them. People have been made to feel guilty and selfish for eating the very foods their DNA craves. Our DNA knows exactly what we need, and ignoring it leads to obesity, disease, and early death.

Let's turn to the farm for some common sense. When a farmer wants to fatten up a cow or pig, what does he feed it? Bacon, butter, and egg yolks, right? That would make perfect sense based on what doctors tell us to avoid when we're trying to lose weight. Umm, no, that wouldn't work at all. It would be very expensive, and the farmer's animals would become leaner, not fatter. When a farmer wants to fatten up livestock as quickly and cheaply as possible, he feeds them starches and carbohydrates as aggressively as the animal can stand it. The feed is usually a combination of corn and grain. If a doctor went to the farm and told the farmer that feeding his cows whole grains and corn would be a great way to help the cows lower their cholesterol and lose weight, he would be justifiably laughed off the farm.

When a farmer wants to cause a goose's liver to become as fatty as possible (pâté is made from the fatty livers of geese), he force-feeds the goose lard and tallow, right? Apparently, that's what a doctor would recommend to the farmer. No, the farmer force-feeds corn to the goose with a plastic tube, a not-very-nice process known as *gavage.* If your doctor has told you that you're developing fatty liver disease because you've been eating too much fat, I hope you're starting to see the silliness of this lie. To fatten up any animal, you feed it large amounts of corn and grain, but somehow, magically, you fatten up humans by feeding them fat? That "logic" doesn't make sense.

THE RESEARCH

You would expect, given how often this medical lie has been and is repeated, that there must be hundreds of medical studies showing beyond all doubt that eating fat makes you fat. In fact, there are no studies showing this to be the case, and there are multiple large studies showing the exact opposite to be true. We expect doctors and experts to think about and study everything, but they don't. Doctors ought to question everything and believe nothing until it has been proven by meaningful medical research. However, when we remember that busy doctors are human, it's understandable that they have believed this medical lie and repeated it because it seemed so self-evident and had been championed by every leading medical authority. It just didn't seem worth the time and study needed to prove or disprove it.

This lie originally gained real traction with the publication of the Seven Countries Study by Dr. Ancel Keys, who started collecting data in 1956 in Yugoslavia and finally published his study in 1978. The deeply flawed (some would say dishonest) study appeared to show that eating saturated fat was linked to rising cholesterol levels in the blood, which would then lead to heart disease. Dr. Keys collected data from twenty-two different countries, but when he published the study, it mysteriously contained data from only seven of those countries, hence its name. Are you wondering why Dr. Keys didn't publish his data from all twenty-two countries? Can you guess? The reason, I kid you not, was because the data from the other countries showed that eating fat either had no effect on the rate of heart disease or actually protected the eater from heart disease. So, the data from those countries was intentionally left out, and suddenly every expert, even the federal government, was telling us that saturated fat had been proven bad for our hearts.

Why did the government get involved, you ask? Dr. Keys had received grants of $200,000 a year from the U.S. Public Health Service. Evidently, they needed to show some results after spending all that money. It quickly became clear to doctors in the United States that unless they wanted to be laughed at, left behind, or worse, they had better climb on board the eat-low-fat, cholesterol-is-bad train. Researchers on the subject began accepting the Seven Countries Study as fact and started doing research—not to retest Dr. Keys's theory but to prove subtheories that were all tainted with the assumption that the Seven Countries Study was proven truth. These studies did some suspect things, like lumping saturated fats and trans fats into the same category, which is an obvious flaw that provides meaningless conclusions when it comes to human nutrition. Trans fats (such as margarine and shortening) are most certainly bad for your health. Lumping them in with saturated fats tainted the research and made the conclusions misleading and dishonest. Only in recent years has more honest research been conducted and published. I discuss Dr. Keys and his study in more detail in Chapter 5.

THE TAKE-HOME

Medical science and doctors are sometimes wrong. Thankfully, they're usually just a little wrong, not completely wrong. However, in this case, it looks like doctors were (and for the most part still are) completely wrong. They're giving you exactly the wrong advice on the subject of nutrition, fat, and health. Telling you to cut down the amount of saturated fat you eat as a way of losing weight and avoiding heart disease won't have the effect most doctors expect. It will remove many tasty things from your diet but result in no meaningful weight loss or decrease in heart disease risk. With the obesity epidemic in our culture, we need to focus on dietary and lifestyle changes that lead to real improvements in our weight and waistlines. Dr. Keys must be taken down from his demigod status and recognized for what he was.

He was someone who wanted to do great things and help humankind. He was also a man who made a horrendous mistake that then became one of the biggest medical lies of all time. He cherry-picked the data he would publish in his flawed study, and he evidently didn't have the courage to admit that his research findings were flawed and had disproved his hypothesis. Most other experts at the time accepted his study without the critical thought they were duty-bound to apply to it, and they parroted his misleading results to the world. The pharmaceutical industry smelled a few billion dollars to be made and jumped into the research wholeheartedly. We shouldn't be surprised that every research study paid for by Big Pharma has found that more and more people should take cholesterol pills and eat less fat. The companies' continued financial success depended on proving this.

Your brain and nerves are made largely of fat and cholesterol. Without the fat in our cell membranes, life as we know it wouldn't be possible, neither would the signaling that occurs between the cells that make up our bodies. We have known this to be medical fact for decades, so I'm still unclear as to why Dr. Keys's study had the huge effect it did on doctors and medical practice. Even to this day, for a doctor to suggest that eating fat is anything but bad is shocking to most people, and especially to most other doctors. When I tell patients that eating fat won't make them fat, as I routinely do, the usual expression is one of shock or disbelief. *(Wait, what did he just say?)* Never in their lives have they heard that phrase before. It flies in the face of every shred of nutritional advice they've ever received from their doctors, their neighbors, and their parents.

I tell them to go home, look in the mirror, and repeat ten times, "Eating fat won't make me fat, but eating sugars and starches will." Usually, that helps them begin to wrap their heads around this new way of thinking. It also allows them to start to think logically about diet and weight loss. Our ancestors never left behind available fat. It was usually the first thing they ate. We should copy their behavior and honor our DNA by eating good fats often.

A hundred years ago, everyone cooked with animal fats like lard and tallow. At that time, heart attacks were unheard of in patients younger than seventy. Obesity was very rare. I often ask patients in their seventies and eighties how many fat kids were in their first-grade class. The answer is always either one or none. Now that we cook everything in vegetable/seed oils and lard is a dirty word, childhood obesity is rampant, and heart attack and stroke are the leading causes of death. It's becoming all too common for people to have their first heart attack in their forties or fifties. Go to the average first-grade class these days and look at the kids who've never eaten anything cooked in lard. Forty percent of children are obese. You think there might be a connection? Here is a hint: A researcher went back over *all* of Dr. Keys's research and found that sugar consumption was much more correlated to heart disease than fat consumption, which means that sugar consumption was much more likely to be the cause of heart disease than fat consumption. The relationship between sugar consumption and heart disease risk existed in all twenty-two countries, not just the seven countries Dr. Keys included in his publication.

If your doctor tells you that the key to losing weight is to eat less fat and exercise more, get up, politely walk out of the interview, and find another doctor. There is probably no hope for him. This one statement, perhaps more than any other a doctor can make, tells you all you need to know about how current this doctor is with his reading and how active he is with his thinking. *Eating fat makes you fat* is the statement of a lazy, unthinking doctor. It's not the statement of someone who has done the work to stay current to be able to give you the correct advice. There are regular individuals who make YouTube videos with better nutrition advice than you can get in the average doctor's office. Doctors have ignored good diet and proper nutrition, both vital to health and long life, for too long. If your doctor doesn't give you real, useful diet and nutrition advice, then get it elsewhere.

DO AS I DO

I include plenty of fat in my diet. Sometimes I eat so much fat that it freaks out my lunch partners. I have found that eating fat to my heart's content helps keep my weight under control and my lab results within normal limits. My body seems to love fat, and it runs much better on fat as fuel. I put grass-fed butter in my coffee and on almost everything else. Egg yolks are now my favorite part of the egg (back in my fat-assed, dumb-doctor days, I would eat only the whites). Bacon is no longer a stranger to my plate.

HOMEWORK

There is so much good information about how healthy good-fat-consumption is that I'm recommending three books, not just two. After reading these books, you will be as smart as any doctor when it comes to the health consequences of eating good fats.

BOOK: *Eat the Yolks* by Liz Wolfe, NTP (2014)

This entertaining book explains in plain words the somewhat complicated story of how fat and cholesterol became dirty words in modern medicine.

BOOK: *The Big Fat Surprise: Why Butter, Meat & Cheese Belong in a Healthy Diet* by Nina Teicholz, MA (2014)

This excellent book is full of studies, citations, and common sense that destroy the myths that red meat, fat, and cholesterol are bad for humans in any way.

BOOK: *Eat Fat, Get Thin: Why the Fat We Eat Is the Key to Sustained Weight Loss and Vibrant Health* by Mark Hyman, MD (2016)

One of the few doctors in the know, Dr. Hyman explains all the ways that eating fat is good for you.

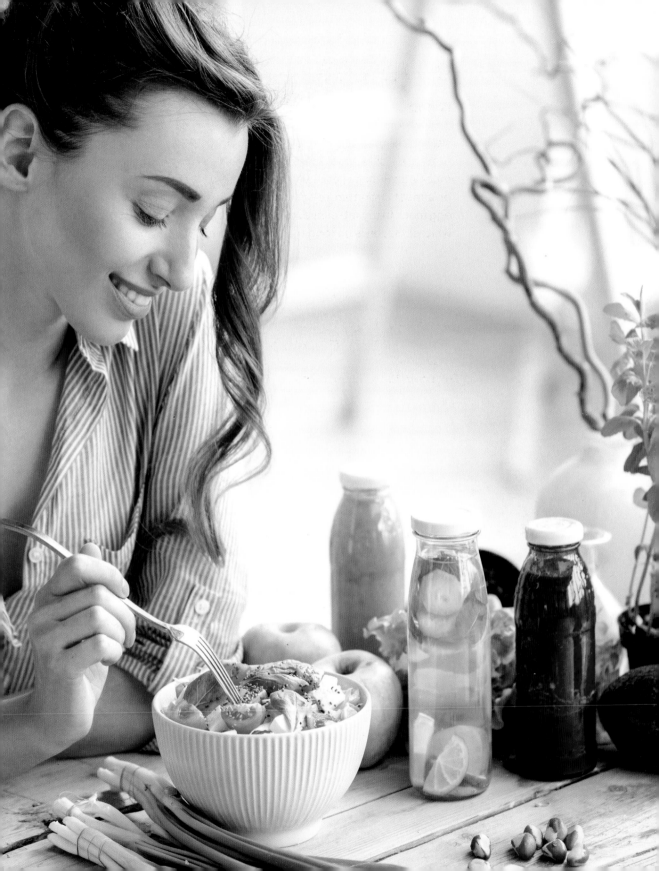

Chapter 4

YOUR BONES DESERVE BETTER

" The reason doctors are
so dangerous is that they
believe in what they
are doing.

—Robert Mendelsohn

"

THE LIE

Drinking milk is good for you and helps keep your bones strong.

WHY YOU SHOULD CARE

You want to eat and drink only what is good for you. If milk is indeed healthy and good for your bones, then drink up. If it is not healthy—but is bad for your bones, as some studies show—then you should avoid it.

SUPPORT FOR THE LIE

Virtually no research shows that drinking milk strengthens human bones, and there is no research showing a society that consumes dairy on a regular basis has stronger bones or is healthier than one that does not. Without research to back up the health claims for dairy, the mega-corporations producing it spend millions of dollars making slick commercials and ad campaigns ("Got Milk?") to trick you into thinking milk is popular and good for you. Now that dairy farms are big business, we can no longer trust what they tell us about their product.

THE COMMON SENSE

Baby mammals are born small and helpless. To survive, they must grow and gain weight as quickly as possible. The milk of mammals is meant to do one thing very well; it is meant to help infant mammals of that species grow and gain weight quickly. Human beings are the only mammals on the planet who drink milk as adults. No other adult animal does this, unless we humans give it to them. As soon as nonhuman mammals are mature enough to catch and digest other food, they stop drinking their mothers' milk.

If drinking milk in adulthood were truly healthy, then you would think at least one other species on the planet would do it. There would be some sneaky weasel who would steal into the nest of another mammal so it could nurse the nutritious milk from its new mommy. But there is no such animal, even though animals will trick and mimic to get almost every other form of nutritional advantage. The common sense of this lie takes us back to the truism that just because something tastes good doesn't mean you should eat or drink it. I tell patients all the time that I hear crack cocaine is amazingly pleasurable, but that doesn't mean we should run out and try it. This statement usually gets a chuckle, as well as a look of understanding.

Milk is the perfect food for babies of the same species as the source that's providing it but is only a tolerably good food for baby mammals of other species. It is well known that milk from different species has different percentages of fat, protein, and other nutrients uniquely tweaked to be the perfect food for babies of that species. Milk from cows is ideally suited as food for young calves but is not a great food for humans. There are much better sources of nutrition for adult humans than milk from another animal.

THE RESEARCH

Recent research shows that drinking milk can weaken bones rather than strengthening them. The countries with the highest dairy consumption have the highest rates of osteoporosis. Countries whose populations drink the most milk have higher rates of hip fractures as they age than countries whose populations drink much less milk. Read those two sentences again and let them sink in.

Studies show we get plenty of calcium from our diet if we eat lots of organic whole foods. Leafy green vegetables are excellent sources of absorbable calcium. They do not have the inflammatory sugars and proteins contained in milk or the other chemicals that are added to milk (either accidentally or on purpose).

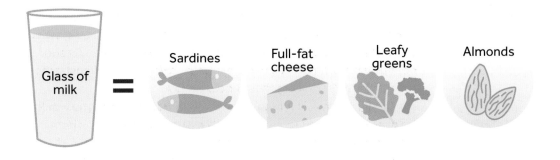

Glass of milk = Sardines | Full-fat cheese | Leafy greens | Almonds

Most of the time, when the calcium contents of two different foods are compared, they are listed by the cup, which can be misleading. A much better way to compare the calcium levels in different foods is to compare them by the calorie. When compared to 100 calories' worth of other foods, 100 calories' worth of milk is revealed to be a very poor source of calcium. In addition, only about one-third of the calcium in milk is absorbable by the human body; the remainder is filtered from your blood by your kidneys and excreted in your urine.

Research is beginning to show that we don't need as much daily calcium as was once believed. An excess of calcium can lead to other problems, including heart artery disease (but not kidney stones!). Cow's milk available in stores does not naturally contain useful amounts of vitamin D; it is added to the milk during processing. The amount of vitamin D added to the milk you find in the grocery is only enough to keep humans from developing rickets. It's not nearly enough to optimize bone and hormonal health. Thus, milk is also a very poor source of vitamin D.

THE TAKE-HOME

When I was a high school student and playing basketball and football, I would drink almost a gallon of milk every day. My teenager brain just knew that this had to be healthy and would make me be a better athlete. I was a decent athlete during my high school years, but I doubt the milk had much to do with it. However, the milk likely had something to do with the chronic allergies, dandruff, and acne I suffered. I could have made much better choices, but I was a high school kid and didn't know much. The television commercials that promoted milk had brainwashed my entire family. The billion-dollar dairy industry spends millions promoting ads on TV and in magazines and millions more lobbying the federal government to make sure that the USDA keeps milk in its misleading MyPlate model (www.choosemyplate.gov/MyPlate).

I think milk is delicious. I would drink it if I could find any research or reasons to convince me that it's healthy, but no meaningful research shows that dairy products are healthy daily choices for food or drink. I often tell my patients that if you are going to drink a dairy product, then please drink heavy (whipping) cream. It has much less milk sugar and fewer of the inflammatory proteins, casein, and whey.

The worst dairy choice of all is skim milk. With all the fat removed, skim milk is an unsatisfying, high-sugar/inflammatory-protein drink that serves no nutritional purpose whatsoever—unless you want to gain weight quickly. The fat in milk is not the culprit of weight gain, as most people and doctors believe. The real culprits are the sugar and inflammatory proteins in the milk.

Today's milk is a heavily processed food. It has been pasteurized and homogenized to the point that it no longer resembles its original self, except for being white. There are multiple problems with the milk production process, which are the subject of numerous books and documentaries. The people with the strongest bones in the world just *don't* drink milk. One large study found that women who drink two to three glasses of milk daily have a higher fracture risk than women who drink less than one glass a day. Another study found that men who drink two or more glasses of milk daily had higher rates of prostate cancer than men who drink less milk. The list goes on and on.

I find it sad that most doctors only halfheartedly encourage mothers to breastfeed their infants the perfect milk that's made for infant humans but wholeheartedly bully the same mother into giving that same child multiple daily servings of cow's milk in later years. You can barely find a doctor who will take a firm, vocal stand saying breast milk is the perfect food for infants and is infinitely better than formula. However, you can line up doctors around the block who tell you that cow's milk is a great food for us at any age, which is another example of the upside-down circus called modern medicine.

There is an argument to be made that raw, organic milk from cows, goats, and other animals might be a healthier food for adults to drink than processed cow's milk. Although organic and unprocessed, these milks are still a concentrated source of milk sugars and proteins. This is an example of assuming that something that's less bad for you is the same as something that's good for you.

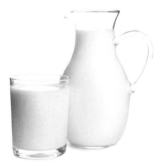

My concern with drinking milk as an adult is threefold.

As I mentioned earlier, if drinking milk as an adult mammal was a smart strategy, you would think other species would have discovered this good source of nutrition in all the thousands of years we've been on this planet. Animals are expert at adapting to things that increase their chances of survival, so you'd think some species would have made use of another animal's milk if it were such a great idea.

Many people are lactose intolerant and can't drink milk at all, so obviously it is bad for them.

Even people who don't suffer from lactose intolerance often have allergic symptoms after drinking milk. I suffered from severe chronic allergies until I stopped drinking milk. Now I never have allergic reactions. I've had multiple patients who suffered from allergies, acid reflux, or acne report that their symptoms improved after they've stopped drinking milk.

There have been times in human history when nutrition was very scarce. During those times, drinking milk was a better alternative than starving. The nutrition in milk has kept many people alive during times of famine. However, in today's time of plenty (at least in most of the Western world), there are much better sources of nutrition than milk. If you love milk and your body can tolerate it, then enjoy it occasionally as a treat. But you should no longer be deluded into thinking that processed milk is a health food. It's not good for your bones or any other part of you. Milk does not do a body good.

DO AS I DO

Drinking milk is a thing of the past for me. I avoid all liquid dairy and would never touch skim milk. I put heavy cream in my coffee, but I never use lower-fat versions of liquid dairy. My weight and mental clarity are much better because I avoid liquid dairy. The dandruff, allergies, and acid reflux I suffered in the past are gone now that I avoid milk. As a result, I will never drink milk again. I get plenty of calcium from the leafy greens and fish that I eat. Because I don't live near the equator and I work mostly indoors, I take a daily vitamin D supplement.

HOMEWORK

The paradigm that milk does a body good is so deeply mired in the subconscious of most doctors and patients that you should probably do a little more reading on the subject if you're still undecided.

BOOK: *Whitewash: The Disturbing Truth About Cow's Milk and Your Health* by Joseph Keon and John Robbins (2010)

This book takes a truthful look at how milk is produced and how our bodies react to it. There are also several documentaries on the Internet about Big Dairy and its questionable practices.

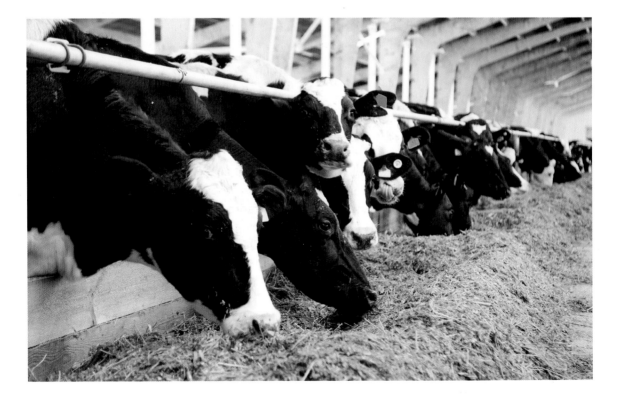

Chapter 5

IS CHOLESTEROL REALLY YOUR ENEMY?

"

It doesn't matter how
beautiful your theory is,
it doesn't matter how
smart you are.
If it doesn't agree with
experiment, it's wrong.

—Richard Feynman

THE LIE

High cholesterol levels in your blood are dangerous and increase your risk of heart attack. You should eat less saturated fat and take cholesterol medicine if your cholesterol level is above normal.

WHY YOU SHOULD CARE

Decreasing the risk of a heart attack should be important to all of us. No one wants to have a heart attack, and we all do whatever it takes to prevent having one. All we need to know is what actually leads to increased risk of heart attacks, and what we need to do to prevent them. If you're taking an expensive, potentially dangerous pill every day to lower your cholesterol and thus prevent a heart attack, you want that pill to do what it's advertised to do, which is to lower your risk of having a heart attack. If, on the other hand, high cholesterol levels don't increase heart attack risk, then let's all shake hands and have some bacon.

SUPPORT FOR THE LIE

Hundreds of research studies, thousands of television commercials, and billions of dollars have been used to convince everyone that high cholesterol is a serious problem for which you need a daily pill (or two). Virtually every expert and organization acts as if this is a no-brainer; they act like you would be a fool not to want to lower your cholesterol. The cholesterol level considered to be normal has been reduced several times over the years. With each decrease, the number of patients who "needed" to take cholesterol medication increased. At one time, doctors considered a total cholesterol level under 300 to be just fine. But then new research (both directly and indirectly funded by Big Pharma) found that level to be much too high and lowered the upper limit of normal to 250, then 240; now we are told that it should be less than 200. Once studies funded by Big Pharma recommend lowering the upper limit of normal low enough, every single human on the planet will meet the criteria for taking a daily cholesterol pill. Obviously, Big Pharma is eager to fund more of these studies.

THE COMMON SENSE

This embarrassing lie, an awful example of medical research and medical science gone wrong, should make patients question every word coming out of their doctors' mouths. Neither common sense nor meaningful research has ever been allowed to play much of a part in this controversial subject.

The common sense concerning this lie is much different from what doctors and the media have taught us. Cholesterol is essential for all animal life. Almost every single cell in your body produces it. Cholesterol makes up at least a third of the cell membrane of every one of your cells. Without cholesterol, none of the cells in your body, including those making up your heart and brain, would function properly. Your body also uses cholesterol as the framework molecule to make vitamin D and all of your sex hormones.

Never so completely has the practice of medicine been hijacked, brainwashed, and made to do the bidding of Big Pharma as when it comes to the cholesterol theory and the medications that lower cholesterol levels. The retelling of this lie is so unbelievable that I won't blame you one bit if you doubt what I say here and must confirm it for yourself. I encourage you to verify the information I tell you about this lie (and all the others).

THE RESEARCH

Scientists have known for more than one hundred years that the human body needs fat and cholesterol to create and repair healthy brain and nervous tissue. In fact, each day your body uses cholesterol for hundreds of different repair processes. However, in the 1950s, that fellow I discussed earlier, Ancel Keys, published the Seven Countries Study. Everyone back then respected Dr. Keys as an honest, intelligent expert. Therefore, when his study showed that eating fat and cholesterol raised a person's cholesterol level and increased that person's chance of having a heart attack, everyone believed him. What no one suspected was that this trusted doctor had manipulated the data he collected, either consciously or unconsciously, to show the outcome he desired. He removed the data that contradicted what he was trying to prove.

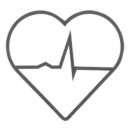

You'll remember that Keys collected data from twenty-two countries. However, he named it the Seven Countries Study.

He simply didn't include the data from the countries that didn't support his theory in his final report. No, I'm not joking. Keys really did that, and the medical community, which evidently was itching for some medical enemy to fight at the time, immediately jumped on the cholesterol-is-bad bandwagon. Butter, eggs, and some meats were vilified based on no research other than this one huge lie told by Dr. Keys.

Some experts disagreed with Dr. Keys and his study findings. However, professional peer pressure and the federal government soon silenced them. Once the cholesterol theory was officially accepted, everyone started trying to cash in on ways to lower patients' cholesterol levels. A great deal of research focused on ways to lower cholesterol. No further research was conducted to confirm Dr. Keys's findings or to try to reproduce them.

In 2015, the USDA Dietary Guidelines Committee Report stated very plainly, "Previously, the Dietary Guidelines for Americans recommended that cholesterol intake be limited to no more than 300 mg/day. The 2015 guidelines will not bring forward this recommendation because available evidence shows no appreciable relationship between consumption of dietary cholesterol and serum cholesterol, consistent with the conclusions of the AHA/ACC report. Cholesterol is not a nutrient of concern for over-consumption." If your eyes just widened in disbelief, you might want to read that again. *NOT A NUTRIENT OF CONCERN FOR OVER-CONSUMPTION!!!* Has your doctor told you this yet? I sure hope so, but I fear it will be you who must tell him.

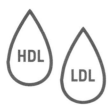

A Japanese study published in the *Annals of Nutrition and Metabolism* in 2015 reported that high cholesterol does not lead to heart disease and protects against many illnesses, including cancer. This study found an inverse relationship between all-cause mortality and cholesterol levels. What does that mean? It means that the higher your cholesterol level, the less likely you are to die from any cause. Yes, you read that right. Very low cholesterol levels are associated with an increased risk of dying. As soon as you finish cursing and throwing things, please come back, and I'll explain why you have been told this medical lie so many times by your doctor and media outlets of every kind.

To this day, Dr. Keys's original flawed work is cited in research studies and the media as if it proves anything other than that humans are flawed and imperfect creations, always capable of making mistakes. Most regular doctors have never heard of Ancel Keys and cannot quote from his study. However, they will repeat, parrot-like, his made-up findings as truth and expect you to follow their recommendations. Research has recently shown that elderly people with the highest cholesterol levels have better memories and less dementia than those with lower cholesterol levels. So, could we doctors have been causing higher levels of dementia in elderly patients by lowering their cholesterol levels with medicine?

Only time and research will tell. More and more, research is showing that a high intake of saturated fats (butter, egg yolks, bacon) has little if any negative effect on heart disease rates. I predict we will continue to find that saturated fats in our diet are not negative but are indeed vital to the function of multiple organs and body systems, the most important being the brain and its memory. Most doctors know that the human brain can burn glucose as energy. However, many doctors have forgotten that the brain also can burn selected fats as energy. Some progressive doctors are starting to believe that the dementia epidemic could be at least partially treated or prevented by increasing fat intake among the elderly and perhaps even by stopping elderly patients' cholesterol medicine (statins).

THE TAKE-HOME

In 1961, Dr. Keys appeared on the cover of *Time* magazine. The associated article described how dietary fat had been *proven* to cause high cholesterol, which led to increased rates of heart disease. For the next fifty years, doctors and patients frantically tried to lower cholesterol levels with a pill, or two, or even three.

However, by 2014, butter was on the cover of *Time*. Yes, butter. The accompanying article was about how medical science had gotten everything wrong for decades; fat and cholesterol in your diet have no effect whatsoever on cholesterol levels or heart disease. It took fifty-plus years for enough thoughtful researchers, doctors, and curious laypeople to topple the shrine erected to the cholesterol theory. What was odd about this medical lie (and also awe-inspiring) is that many non-medical people had somehow gotten wise to it before the media had even started talking about it. Alternative medical thinkers and individual patients had out-thought the medical elite. They somehow knew that statin pills were more dangerous than the cholesterol levels these pills were supposed to treat.

When I was still a believer in the cholesterol theory, I remember having patients who were afraid of the side effects of cholesterol-lowering medicines and wouldn't take them. I wasn't sure, at the time, why they felt this way, and I was too arrogant at the time to explore their "foolishness." However, they had it figured out. I would try to get them to at least take a very low-dose statin drug, so they could get some "protection." They would feign being allergic to any cholesterol medicine I started them on. As the years passed and I continued to study, I slowly realized that I was doing my patients no favors by prescribing high-dose statin therapy (the most recommended form of cholesterol-lowering medicine). Consequently, I gradually decreased their statin doses with each scheduled refill.

As many of my patients have transitioned from high-dose statin therapy to very low-dose or no-dose statin therapy, there has been no increase in the rate of heart attack in these patients. However, I certainly have noticed a decrease in their muscle aches and stiffness and an increase in their energy levels. Meanwhile, my colleagues were busy prescribing the highest-dose statin therapy their patients could tolerate, despite the published fact that most patients who have a heart attack have a cholesterol level of less than 200. My fellow doctors were busy making Lipitor the bestselling drug in history without preventing heart attacks.

Many doctors today, even though they are beginning to understand that the cholesterol theory of heart disease is flawed, are hesitant to stop their patients' statin medications due to fear of lawsuits and/or medical board consequences. It is truly a shame when doctors are afraid to do the right thing for their patients. If you're on a statin, talk to your doctor about slowly decreasing the dosage. Also, please take a daily dose of coenzyme Q10 (200 mg) along with the statin. Taking coenzyme Q10 can reduce the muscle aches associated with taking a statin, and it's very good for your heart health as well. I wouldn't blame you if you decided to stop taking a statin altogether.

If you feel like I'm tiptoeing around just telling you that taking a statin is stupid, that statins do not protect you from heart attack, and that statins might be hurting you, you're correct. I've already felt the wrath of my medical board for recommending natural alternatives to prescription medications, and thus my attorney is a little gun-shy of me running my mouth too much and incurring another fine, or worse.

I predict that one day, history will look back on the cholesterol theory of heart disease and the statin era of medicine with shame and embarrassment. Medical schools will use this period as an example of how research can go wrong and how Big Pharma can influence medical practice for profit. We doctors let our practices, and the care we give our patients, be hijacked by Big Pharma based on flawed research as we were being bluffed and/or stiff-armed by our medical societies and medical boards to comply, or else.

Shameful practices such as this are a large part of the reason that alternative and homeopathic medicine are making inroads and are starting to be accepted by patients as being effective. I can't blame patients for feeling this way and for trying other alternatives. If what your doctor is recommending is silly and perhaps dangerous, then you're justified in looking elsewhere for advice on preventing heart attacks. We doctors can try to blame the drug-makers and the medical journals for this travesty in modern medicine all we want, but we doctors were signing all those prescriptions.

DO AS I DO

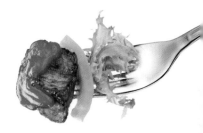

I never give a thought to the cholesterol content of any food I eat. I eat as my ancestors would have eaten thousands of years ago and let my body take care of the rest. Although my diet is cholesterol-filled, my cholesterol levels are always within the normal range.

HOMEWORK

The average doctor is far behind on his homework concerning this lie, so you should do a little homework yourself. Read the following books to become an expert on cholesterol and what it means for your health.

BOOK: *The Great Cholesterol Myth* by Jonny Bowden and Stephen Sinatra, MD (2015)
This book was written by a nutritionist and a cardiologist who teamed up to tease out the truth of this overly complicated subject.

BOOK: *The Cholesterol Myths: Exposing the Fallacy That Saturated Fat and Cholesterol Cause Heart Disease* by Uffe Ravnskov, MD/PhD (2000)
This book includes good information that will make it easy to understand why you shouldn't fear fat and cholesterol.

Chapter 6

WHEAT ISN'T ALL IT'S CRACKED UP TO BE

Does history record any case in which the majority was right?

—Robert A. Heinlein

THE LIE

Wheat is a healthy food that is very good for your body. Everyone should eat multiple servings of whole-wheat foods every day.

WHY YOU SHOULD CARE

We all want to be as healthy as possible, and we get this way only if we eat the healthiest foods and live the healthiest lifestyle. If wheat is good for us, then we should eat it all the time. If, however, it isn't good for us, then we should limit how much of it we eat or avoid eating it at all.

SUPPORT FOR THE LIE

Endorsement of wheat as a health food is akin to a religious belief when it comes to governmental and medical experts who make dietary recommendations. From the USDA's Food Pyramid and newer MyPlate models to the newly minted medical student, everyone passionately tells you that you're not eating enough whole wheat. Doctors admit that a few people with celiac disease should not eat wheat, but they think the majority of people thrive on its nourishment. You will be hard-pressed to find a single authoritative committee or organization that doesn't consider wheat a perfect food. We are told that wheat helps in everything from cancer prevention to weight loss, especially products made with 100 percent whole wheat. You would expect volumes of meaningful research to be available on this subject given the experts' wholehearted endorsement of whole wheat, but you will soon find this to be untrue.

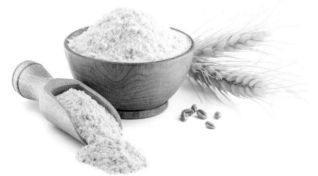

THE COMMON SENSE

At first glance, wheat would seem to be just another plant growing from the dirt. Therefore, it should be safe to eat and nourishing to our bodies unless it contains poison, as some plants do. Because wheat is a plant that comes from the earth, common sense suggests that wheat has the stamp of approval. Applying this same thinking to eating other plants, like castor beans and rhubarb leaves, is soon revealed as folly because they both contain poisons that can sicken or even kill you. Just being a plant doesn't automatically make something healthy for humans.

The wheat that bread is made from today is markedly different from the wheat our great-grandparents' bread was made from. As discussed earlier, another commonsense view is that farmers feed wheat, corn, and other grains to the livestock they want to fatten for market rather than feeding them the grass that cows crave or the fat that supposedly makes humans gain weight. If wheat fattens a cow, it probably fattens humans, too.

THE RESEARCH

There are no meaningful research studies showing that eating wheat, either whole or processed, is good for your body. Just because eating a plant causes no obvious short-term problems doesn't mean it's good for your long-term health. There are research studies that show that whole-grain foods are slightly healthier than foods made with bleached flour. Based on these studies, whole-wheat food is recommended as healthy by the average doctor.

This is another example of the thought-error of declaring something is good for you only because it is less bad than something else. The argument that whole wheat is healthier than processed wheat is exactly like the story about the research study comparing unfiltered and filtered cigarettes that I discuss in Chapter 2. Doctors accept and repeat the lie that wheat is great for human health as self-evident without needing further research.

THE TAKE-HOME

Glycemic Index

Low (less than 15)   Medium (15 – 39)   High (40 or higher)

Fruits

Grapefruit (120g)	25
Apples (120g)	40
Strawberries (120g)	40
Bananas (120g)	47
Peaches, fresh (120g)	56
Kiwifruit (120g)	58
Dates (60g)	62
Watermelon (120g)	80

Vegetables

Spinach (100g)	15
Carrots, raw (80g)	35
Tomato soup (250g)	38
Sweet potato, boiled, (150g)	61
Pumpkin (80g)	66
Potato, mashed (150g)	83

Nuts and Legumes

Cashews (50g)	25
Kidney beans (150g)	29
Black beans (150g)	30
Butter beans (150g)	36
Lentils, canned (150g)	42
Split pea soup (250g)	60
Black bean soup (250g)	64
Broad beans (80g)	79

Snacks and Sweets

Hummus (30g)	6
Corn chips (50g)	42
Snickers (60g)	43
Blueberry muffin (60g)	50
Honey, pure (25g)	58
Sugar, table (25g)	65
French fries (150g)	75
Doughnuts, cake (47g)	76
Pretzels (30g)	83

Grains, Breads, and Cereals

Barley (150g)	22
Chickpeas (150g)	36
Bran cereal (30g)	43
Instant noodles (180g)	52
Taco shells (20g)	68
Bagel, white (70g)	69
White bread (30g)	70
Waffles (35g)	76
Corn flakes (30g)	79

Dairy and Dairy Alternatives

Skim milk (250g)	32
Soy milk (250g)	43
Tofu, frozen dessert, nondairy (50g)	115

Meat

Beef	0
Chicken	0
Fish	0

The *glycemic index* of bread, whether whole wheat or not, is higher than that of table sugar. This means that eating two slices of bread will make your blood sugar increase faster than eating a spoonful of pure sugar. This fact alone should make everyone reconsider how healthy wheat is. Glucose spikes and the accompanying insulin spikes appear to be the root cause of obesity and multiple other chronic diseases. Please doubt my word and research these facts for yourself. Some experts argue that *glycemic load* is more important than glycemic index, but, even if true, that doesn't make the glycemic index of a food unimportant. The great majority of my patients express disbelief the first time I tell them that eating wheat is slowly turning them into fat diabetics. Only after I repeat this several times and explain the reasoning behind it and after the patients have lost weight by stopping or slowing their wheat intake do they begin to believe and understand that the "facts" about wheat that they thought they knew were just part of another medical lie.

The truth is that everything from cataracts in the eye to arthritis in the knees, from high triglyceride levels to high blood sugar levels, are largely caused by eating multiple daily servings of foods that contain wheat. It appears that eating wheat causes these problems just as quickly as (or even quicker than) eating a jelly donut. You can easily find the few minerals and vitamins in wheat products (white bread is virtually devoid of nutrients) in other, healthier foods that have more acceptable glycemic indexes. Why do you think wheat is pushed as aggressively as it is by Big Food and by the medical experts it funds?

Big Food (the huge corporations that profit from manufacturing and marketing food products) can make anything and everything, from pizza crusts to cookies, with inexpensive wheat flour. Given all the big-government subsidies given to wheat producers, they can make it very, very cheaply, thus leading to increased profits. What a hugely profitable run Big Food has had by marketing and selling wheat as a health food. It's a shame that this wheat doesn't live up to all the hype.

The wheat contained in all the food products on store shelves today is very different from the wheat of our ancestors. Today's wheat is a semi-dwarf hybrid wheat that was starting to be bred in the 1960s, and it's become the only type of wheat in products on today's grocery shelves. It has a much higher gluten content than older varieties of wheat, such as einkorn. Many experts are increasingly finding that this hybrid wheat leads to increases in inflammation both in patients with documented celiac disease and in normal patients who don't have this condition.

The gluten and other proteins in today's hybrid wheat seem to contribute to gut inflammation and leakiness, both of which can lead to body-wide inflammation and possibly even to autoimmune conditions such as hypothyroidism and lupus. I've had several patients tell me of enjoying increased weight loss and mental clarity, among many other benefits, after greatly decreasing wheat in their diets. Until further meaningful research explores these connections, it's best to minimize wheat in your diet, even if you do not have celiac disease. Two good general rules are to avoid any product that comes from a factory in a cardboard box and to avoid all bread, crackers, and pasta. I know some of you are feeling anguish at the very thought of eliminating these foods from your diet, almost as if you are addicted to them or something.

Speaking of addiction, research has uncovered convincing evidence that wheat contains substances that partially activate the opiate receptor in the brain (which causes activation of the pleasure centers) and have addictive potential. Several experts in the field consider substances in wheat food products to be habit-forming, which could explain why we want to eat every two to three hours when we're trying to live on a low-fat whole-grain diet. Many people find that they strongly crave these products a few days after they stop eating them. Many fail in their diet attempts and go back to eating as they did before. We need to do further study on this subject, but it's quite possible that the craving you have for baked goods is an actual addiction.

A newer drug being used to assist weight loss, called naltrexone, works by blocking the pleasure receptors in the brain. It can prevent the food cravings and thus lead to weight loss. It takes five to fourteen days to break the cravings associated with wheat after you stop eating it. After that, you can pretty much take it or leave it. I suggest that you leave it. I've had many patients tell me they felt tired and achy for two weeks after stopping grains. Many of them compare it to a time they tried to stop caffeine. However, once they pass the two-week mark, they feel better both mentally and physically, and the weight loss begins.

DO AS I DO

These days, I rarely eat any wheat at all. If pizza is the only choice available at a meal, I eat the toppings and leave the crust behind. I order meatballs and the sauce and have the server hold the noodles (which seems to upset servers for some reason). My health and weight have responded remarkably to this way of eating.

I went from being a fat-assed doctor who told my patients to lose weight to a doctor who leads by example when it comes to his waistline. Sometimes I do eat an occasional treat of something containing wheat, but I am fully aware it is just that: a treat. It isn't real food for nourishing my body.

HOMEWORK

It's apparently going to take most doctors another decade or two to catch up on their reading when it comes to wheat and its negative effects on human health. Therefore, you can help your doctor start to catch up on this important information after reading these two excellent works.

BOOK: *Wheat Belly: Lose the Wheat, Lose the Weight, and Find Your Path Back to Health* by William Davis, MD (2014)

Dr. Davis does an excellent job of breaking down the arguments and exposing the flawed science that has fooled modern medicine about this topic.

BOOK: *Grain Brain: The Surprising Truth about Wheat, Carbs, and Sugar–Your Brain's Silent Killers* by David Perlmutter, MD (2013)

Dr. Perlmutter presents overwhelming reasoning for why you should get wheat out of your life, your belly, and your brain.

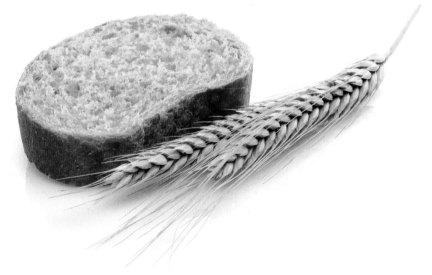

Chapter 7

THE PYRAMID OF FOOD LIES

> # 66
>
> **Often the less there is to justify a traditional custom, the harder it is to get rid of it.**
>
> —Mark Twain
>
> 99

THE LIE

The USDA Food Pyramid and MyPlate models offer the healthiest way to make food choices. If you follow them, you will have better health.

WHY YOU SHOULD CARE

The logical conclusion is that the obesity and diabetes epidemics that our society is suffering from must be directly related to our diets. Choosing the wrong foods on a daily basis can result in you being overweight and sick, or worse. Along with not smoking, making smart food choices is the most important daily health decision you make. If the Food Pyramid and MyPlate guidelines are good for our weight and our health, then we should follow them. If the Food Pyramid and MyPlate guidelines are good only for the profit margins of Big Agriculture and Big Food, then we should look elsewhere for dietary advice.

SUPPORT FOR THE LIE

Many references to expert consensus, as well as several studies with worrisome conclusions that were based on iffy research, are used to support the Food Pyramid and MyPlate food choice guidelines. There is no meaningful research showing that people who adhere to the Food Pyramid or MyPlate models will have healthier body weights or better overall health. The federal government and every expert will, however, tell you to follow the Food Pyramid and MyPlate guidelines.

THE COMMON SENSE

For 99.99 percent of human existence on this planet, humans have been slim, fit, and diabetes-free. We never, as a species, ate the amounts of grains and low-fat dairy that are recommended by the USDA Food Pyramid and MyPlate guidelines. It stands to reason that we should eat as our ancestors did because they survived, thrived, and reproduced from the beginning of their existence to the day you were born. Of course, diets varied from region to region and from season to season, so there is not one single formula that we all must follow. Less important than what you *should* eat is what you *shouldn't* eat.

Some ancestral diets were very plant-heavy, whereas others consisted mainly of animal products. Both sets of ancestors thrived, even though their diets were very different. The few things that none of our ancestors consumed until a few hundred years ago were grains in any quantity, low-fat dairy, and high levels of sugars and processed starches. Our DNA is not yet able to use these products as sustenance for keeping our bodies healthy and lean. Obesity rates have increased steadily since the USDA introduced the Food Pyramid and MyPlate guidelines.

THE RESEARCH

If you want to understand how an agency like the USDA runs, then just Google *food pyramid history*. You will read how Big Food and Big Agriculture got the final say in these guidelines. You also will learn how these corporate giants got to make drastic changes to the Food Pyramid guidelines before those guidelines were published.

For example, Big Food and Big Agriculture companies got to proofread and change some of the guidelines after the nutrition scientists had finished with them but before the public saw them. Keep searching the Internet, and you will have as much trouble as I did finding any research that proves the Food Pyramid or MyPlate system does anything positive for your health. Good luck in your search, and don't be too disappointed with your government and Big Food. You might have done the same thing had you been in their shoes.

THE TAKE-HOME

The USDA Food Pyramid and MyPlate guidelines repeat many medical lies. This pyramid of disease encourages you to eat more starches, more dairy, less fat, fewer veggies, and less meat than you should. The amount of grains (breads, crackers, pasta, cereals, and so on) recommended is ridiculous, and the amount of low-fat dairy recommended is worrisome. As you would expect, healthy fats and salt are demonized. Low-fat and fat-free dairy is pushed as the healthiest choice, whereas healthy fats are lumped in with unhealthy fats and "vegetable" oils.

You should now be asking, "Why would my government publish this sort of thing if it wasn't correct and helpful?" That's a very good question. The answer might surprise or sicken you (or both). When the USDA was designing the Food Pyramid, it initially recommended five servings of grains and five to nine servings of fruit daily. The Pyramid was originally designed by nutrition experts who knew a thing or two about human nutrition. However, as government is prone to do, the USDA let Big Food and Big Agriculture take a look at the suggested Food Pyramid guidelines before publication.

In the end, the government allowed profit-driven corporations to make changes that made the guidelines more acceptable from the viewpoint of the corporations, their boards of directors, and their future profits. When the proposed Food Pyramid came back from the corporations, it had been violated to protect their profits. The guidelines thereafter recommended six to eleven servings of grains (up from five) and only two to three servings of fruit (down from five to nine) daily. Dairy had gotten a section of its own, as if it were a necessary food category for all humans to consume, even though 80 percent of the people on the planet are unable to consume dairy. Also, processed and "junk" foods were lumped in with natural, whole foods in all the guideline sections. The agency that most people assume is watching over their food and their health had perpetrated an embarrassing and worrisome sellout. This is another story that you can research on your own.

For most of our species' existence on this planet, we have been hunter-gatherers and/or nomads. We never raised or ate grains in any meaningful amounts. The grains we grew and ate barely resembled the Big Agriculture wheat of today. Our ancestors always ate the highest-fat part of their meals first. If one of our ancestors had requested something low-fat, he would probably have been stoned to death for stupidity. As our DNA has evolved over the eons, it grew accustomed to certain foods and never had to deal with certain other things that we're now told are "healthy" foods.

If you could go back in time and transport your forty-seventh great-grandfather to the present day, he would most certainly be muscular, lean, alert, and sharp, even in his elder years. If you made him follow the Food Pyramid guidelines (and you would have to make him; he wouldn't do it willingly), he would become fat, sick, and sluggish in less than a year. His DNA would have no idea what to do with all the starches, sugars, and low-fat dairy. Eating those things would put fat on his belly, waist, and butt, as well as inside his liver. It makes sense (since we share the exact same DNA) that the reverse should also be true. If you were to take a modern human (you) back in time and feed him only what his distant ancestors would have eaten, you would change him from fat, sick, and sluggish to muscular, lean, and sharp.

Because the guidelines are not mandatory for most of us, people don't give a lot of thought to the Food Pyramid and MyPlate; however, they should. Even though you might not consult the Food Pyramid and MyPlate guidelines, any institution that prepares food and receives federal funds—like public school cafeterias and most hospital cafeterias—have to follow the guidelines. Our growing children and the sickest among us are often trapped in situations where they have no choice but to eat according to the USDA's Food Pyramid and/or MyPlate guidelines. This is a danger to students and patients, and it's shameful for doctors and nutrition experts to lazily allow this to happen. These experts falsely believe that the USDA is in business to promote health, forgetting that the A in USDA stands for agriculture (Big Agriculture), not health. However, you can choose to eat properly, according the needs of your DNA, and to try to make changes at your local school and hospital. You should start with yourself and your diet first, though.

If your doctor tells you the key to losing weight is to cut back on calories, exercise more, and follow the Food Pyramid or MyPlate guidelines, you should get up, politely walk out of the interview, and find another doctor. Any doctor who says this is revealing a complete absence of thought or effort on his part. Therefore, you probably won't be able to educate him to be your partner in health.

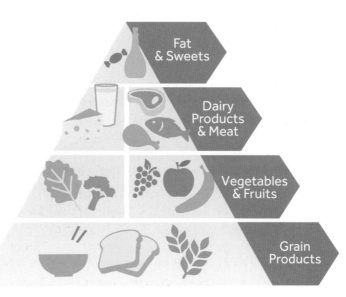

DO AS I DO

I would never punish my body by eating according to the Food Pyramid or MyPlate guidelines. I eat according to my DNA, as my ancestors ate. If I did anything less, it would be a betrayal to both. Of course, I occasionally have a treat that I know is not good for me; we all do that.

With my patients, I use the example of the honey tree. Probably once every year or two, our ancestors would have had the luck to find a bee-filled honey tree and the bravery to attack it. I can picture them lying around in a sleepy sugar coma for days after indulging in this special treat. Occasional indulgences like this aren't harmful, but daily treats can lead to obesity and disease.

HOMEWORK

It seems that some people, and some doctors, just can't shake the belief that *if the federal government says something, then it's the truth.* Because you have only one life and you want it to be a healthy one, I recommend you stop believing big government and read this excellent book.

BOOK: *Death by Food Pyramid: How Shoddy Science, Sketchy Politics and Shady Special Interests Have Ruined Our Health* by Denise Minger (2014)

Denise proves you don't have to be a doctor or researcher to write meaningfully on the topics of nutrition and health. After reading her book, you'll always translate terms such as *government guidelines* and *government recommendations* to what they really mean: *special interest groups came up with this recommendation to benefit their bottom line, not my health.*

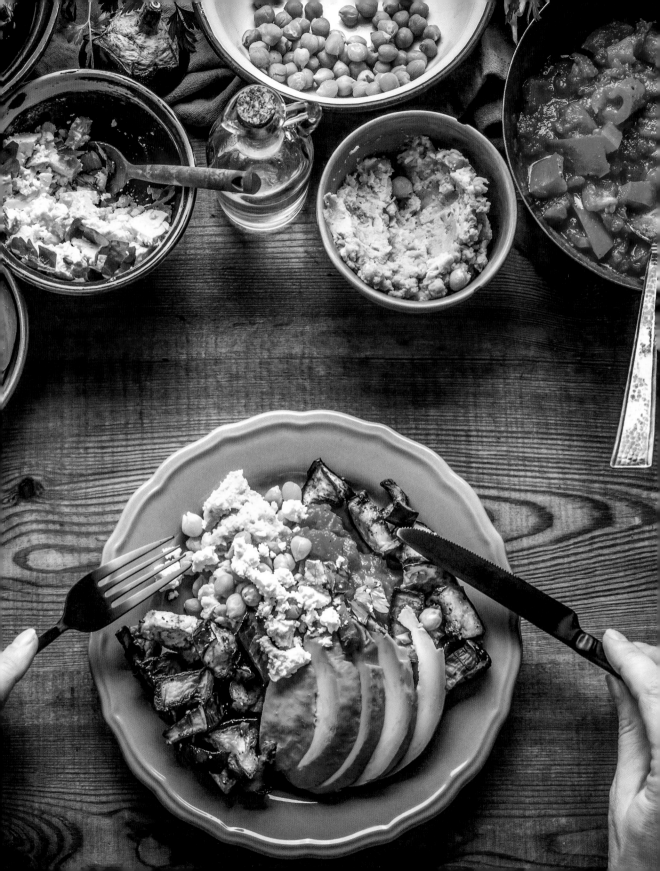

Chapter 8

EXERCISE IS GREAT, BUT IT WON'T HELP MUCH WITH WEIGHT LOSS

I firmly believe that if the whole *materia medica* could be sunk to the bottom of the sea, it would be all the better for mankind and all the worse for the fishes.

—Oliver Wendell Holmes

THE LIE

If you exercise more, you will lose weight.

WHY YOU SHOULD CARE

Being overweight, even a little, is dangerous for your long-term health. It's vital that you know how to spend your time, effort, and money to reach and maintain a healthy weight. If exercise does lead to significant weight loss, then you should do it faithfully, even if you don't enjoy it. If, on the other hand, exercise does little to cause significant weight loss, then you should focus your time, effort, and money elsewhere and stop feeling guilty about not having joined a gym.

SUPPORT FOR THE LIE

Almost every doctor in the world will tell you this medical lie. The doctor will look at you like you're from Mars if you ask to see the research proving it. To doctors who haven't read the research about the futility of exercise with regard to weight loss and who still believe in the *all calories are equal* and *burn more calories than you eat* lies, it seems self-evident that the more you exercise, the more weight you will lose. When we look for research to back up this claim, we come away empty-handed. Expect every doctor and expert to tell you this exercise-to-lose-weight lie and to belittle you if you doubt it. You should also expect every gym, sports equipment manufacturer, and sports clothing manufacturer to tell you this same lie. It is in their financial best interest to do so.

THE COMMON SENSE

Common sense is sometimes wrong; this is why we humans came up with the scientific method; it was scientists' attempt to remove fallible human nature from the equation where important things like scientific conclusions and medical advice were concerned. In the case of this exercise-to-lose-weight lie, it seems to make perfect sense that the more you exercise, the more calories you will burn, and therefore the more weight you will lose. When you eat, you take in calories, right? When you exercise, you burn calories, right? So, if you exercise enough, you should be able to burn off any number of calories you have eaten to create a *calorie deficit*.

It seems like a simple solution. Just join a gym or buy some home exercise equipment, use it daily, and you'll be on your way to a leaner body. This is one of the times we need the scientific method to protect us from our "common sense." This line of reasoning makes so much sense to us that, even though the research shows that exercise is all but useless for weight loss, doctors still repeat this medical lie to their patients all the time.

THE RESEARCH

Research studies uniformly show that exercise is a very poor method of weight loss. More than sixty meaningful studies show very little benefit from exercise as a means of losing weight. As a young doctor, if someone had said those two sentences to me, I would have laughed at them for saying such foolish things; most doctors still would laugh. Please do some research to verify those statements for yourself. Then stop feeling guilty because you hate the treadmill, and focus your money and effort elsewhere.

THE TAKE-HOME

Although it might be hard to convince yourself of this, it has been proven, beyond a doubt, that exercising more is a terrible method for losing weight. You may need to repeat this several times while looking at yourself in the mirror before you believe it. You might need to get up, take this book into the next room, and whack your spouse over the head with it (but not too hard). Tell them to read that sentence aloud and then shut the hell up about hassling you to exercise more! This medical lie is still repeated daily for several reasons: the commonsense issue, money-making opportunities, and our seeming need to use guilt as a motivator.

Common sense is a very useful tool. It helps us figure out the world and all the problems it throws at us on a daily basis. When you drop a ball, you know which direction it will travel, and you also know what will happen when it hits the floor, even if you have never dropped that particular ball before. Common sense gives us hundreds of mental shortcuts that save us time and effort. Sometimes, however, common sense can fool or confuse us, and this medical lie about exercise is one of those times. Even now, you may be reading this with a bit of suspicion, because it seems to make so much sense that exercising more will lead to significant weight loss. Profit-hungry corporations are quick to exploit this error in common sense to make a fortune. The companies do it in both blatant and subtle ways. They probably truly believe this lie themselves. There is money to be made on both sides of the equation. Food companies advertise to associate their unhealthy products with all kinds of sports, whereas gyms and exercise equipment companies cash in by selling you the things you need to use to burn off more calories than you eat.

Imagine that you are in the business of selling granola bars. You know they don't contain much in the way of nutrition, and they contain lots of sugar. Still, they taste so darn good that people are tempted to buy them anyway. How could you help your customers give in to temptation and buy your granola bars? What if you told them all they had to do was burn more calories by exercising more and they could enjoy all the granola bars their bellies desire without any consequences? You could even include a discount coupon in your packaging for the local gym to encourage your customers to exercise more. Your granola bars might take on the image of being health conscious.

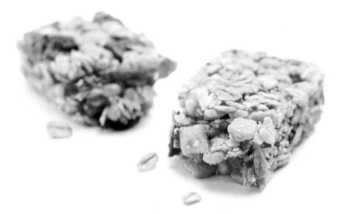

Food and beverage companies have been doing things like this since the 1920s. Ads showed famous athletes drinking a cola after a vigorous ball game or showed children enjoying their treats after coming in from playing outdoors. Food and beverage companies don't want you to know what the research shows about the relationship (or lack thereof) between exercise and weight loss. If you knew without a doubt that no amount of exercise would erase the damage done by eating those granola bars, then you just wouldn't eat them.

Now imagine you're selling sportswear or athletic shoes. How could you take advantage of this error in thinking to make a fortune? You know that almost half of your customers are obese, so all you have to do is help them see that by exercising in your new shoes or your new line of spandex, they will be able to lose weight by burning off all calories from the food and beverages they've consumed. You could have the same athlete who drank the cola after his big game wearing your shoes *during* the game. That would tie everything together. Can you see how companies get in your wallet coming and going? First, you buy the food and beverage because you have plans to exercise more and burn off the calories. You then buy the shoes because you need them so you can run farther and faster to burn off all the calories you've consumed. Companies selling athletic equipment, shoes, clothing, and workout videos don't want you to know about the research because, if you did, you would certainly save your money rather than wasting it on their products.

Guilt can be used in many ways to exploit this error in common sense and lack of knowledge about the true nature of the research. Your doctor might imply that you're to blame for being overweight because you eat too much and don't exercise enough. By doing this, your doctor is relieved of the responsibility of not educating you correctly on how to lose weight, and he places all the blame (guilt) on you because you aren't doing the right things. Advertisers also exploit your sense of guilt. The shoe company shows dedicated models exercising in their shoes. You will look at these ads and feel the guilt in your gut because you'll think, "I'll look like that model if I exercise more." You know you need to buy those shoes and start running today. The granola bar company tries to erase the guilt you should feel from eating their worthless bars by helping you make plans to exercise more in the future to burn off the calories.

You're caught in an endless guilt cycle. You feel guilty for eating the granola bars, and you feel guilty for buying the shoes and not using them as much as you should. To make things worse, your doctor, who should know better, confirms all this guilt by pointing out that your extra weight is all your fault anyway. To add insult to injury, you have a much lighter wallet because you spent all your money on granola bars and shoes! None of this guilt helps you achieve your health goals.

Don't spend your time, effort, or money on hours of exercise for the sole purpose of losing weight, and definitely don't invest in all the shoes, clothing, and gym memberships advertisers tell you are necessary to make exercise successful. Many people spend hours each week slaving away at a gym they hate and spending money on memberships, shoes, and other equipment to help them exercise more. When this doesn't work to help them achieve their goals, they feel guilty for their failure. They are sure that it would have worked if only they had been more dedicated.

Let me be clear about exercise and what it will do for you. It's wonderful for your mind, body, and spirit in hundreds of ways. Exercise will make you healthier and happier (if you're doing exercise you enjoy), but it will not help you lose weight. Many studies show that exercise does everything from decreasing your risk of dementia to building good-looking muscle, so there are plenty of benefits to exercise. But don't spend your time, money, and effort on exercise because you want to lose weight when you'd be better off putting your effort toward strategies that actually work.

If your doctor tells you the key to losing weight is to cut back on calories and to exercise more, politely walk out of the interview and find another doctor. Or you could maybe hand the doctor a copy of this book and tell him he's perpetuating a careless and damaging lie when he tells an overweight patient to exercise more.

DO AS I DO

I'm very active and exercise a lot, but I never, ever "work out." I jump on the trampoline with my kids, cut down trees, lift heavy things on my little farm, and sometimes run really fast. However, I never do any of these things for the purpose of losing weight. I wouldn't join the gym if it were free, and you couldn't pay me to run on a treadmill.

Do what you enjoy. Don't work out; go outside and play! Fun, playful exercise is great for your body, mind, and soul, but you need to look elsewhere for meaningful weight loss. If you truly enjoy running on a treadmill, then, by all means, do it daily. But, don't expect that activity to lead to permanent weight loss.

HOMEWORK

You probably won't get much help from your doctor on this subject. You're better to read the following book and then let your doctor borrow it. He might thank you for helping him to stop mindlessly repeating this medical lie.

BOOK: *The Calorie Myth: How to Eat More, Exercise Less, Lose Weight, and Live Better* by Jonathan Bailor (2015)

This is one of the very best books I have read that explains how food quality, not food and exercise quantity, is the key to meaningful weight loss.

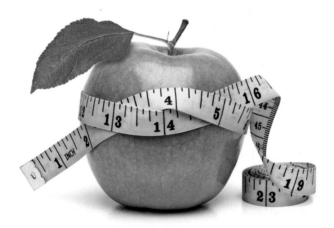

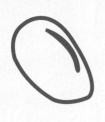

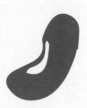

Chapter 9

NUTS AND SEEDS DON'T CAUSE THIS PROBLEM

The specialist is too commonly hypertrophied in one direction and atrophied in all the rest.

—Martin H. Fisher

THE LIE

Eating popcorn, nuts, and seeds will either cause diverticulitis or cause your diverticulitis to flare up.

WHY YOU SHOULD CARE

Diverticulosis is a condition that occurs when small pouches form and push outward through apparent weak spots in the wall of the large intestine. The pouches often develop in the lower part of the large intestine. They are common in individuals who eat a Western diet and are older than forty. Most people with diverticulosis do not have symptoms or problems. However, some people have attacks of diverticulitis (inflammation or infection in those small pouches) that can be quite severe. If eating nuts and seeds causes flare-ups of diverticulitis, then you should avoid eating those foods. However, nuts and seeds are very nutritious. Therefore, if it's a medical lie that nuts and seeds cause flare-ups, then everyone with diverticulosis should enjoy them for their taste and many health benefits.

SUPPORT FOR THE LIE

There is no scientific support for this medical lie. I couldn't find one large, reputable study that supports this statement. *None.* As I reflect on this, it makes me worry about doctors who repeat lies like this with no supporting research because the lie appeals to our common sense.

THE COMMON SENSE

Common sense is once again behind how people—even doctors— widely believe and repeat this medical lie. It seems to make good common sense that if you have small pouches in the lining of your large intestine, then eating tiny things like seeds might increase the risk of diverticulitis. It also makes sense that one of these little seeds could clog the opening of one of the pouches and cause problems because clogging the opening could cause the pouch to become inflamed or infected (which is the definition of diverticulitis).

THE RESEARCH

One very large, well-done research study shot this medical lie in the head years ago. It was published in *JAMA (Journal of the American Medical Association),* and it should have been required reading for every doctor in the country. However, doctors and news sources refuse to let this lie die the death it deserves. This study included thousands of participants, and it showed, without doubt, that some foods do increase your risk of getting diverticulitis. However, seeds, nuts, and popcorn are not on the list of problem foods. The patients in the study who reported eating the most nuts, seeds, and popcorn were the least likely to get diverticulitis. Yes, you read that right.

This lie is very revealing in that it demonstrates that doctors don't need any medical research to believe fervently in a medical lie and to repeat it to their patients. Very good doctors thoughtlessly repeat this lie to patients who would really benefit from the nutrition in nuts and seeds. If doctors would become familiar with the study in *JAMA,* they'd know that the nuts and seeds probably protect patients from having bouts of diverticulitis.

THE TAKE-HOME

Nuts and seeds are some of the healthiest foods you can eat. The nutrients and fiber they contain are great for your health. When I was in my residency training and first taught the lie that nuts and seeds are a problem, I was suspicious, but, as is typical of a resident, I was so tired and busy I had no time to research the information. This lie was reinforced many times in my training by experts in the field. It was only after I completed residency and started my practice that I had time to look into the research behind this lie. As is often the case in medical practice, a patient must suffer for a doctor to learn.

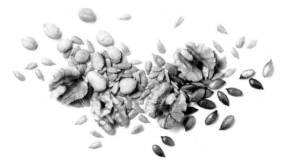

I had sent a patient who was having severe bouts of diverticulitis to see a gastroenterologist (a specialist in the stomach and intestines) in a nearby metropolitan medical center. The patient went to see the specialist and returned to see me a few weeks later. When I walked into the exam room, my patient was anxious about telling me what he had learned because he feared I would be offended. He knew I encouraged all my patients to eat a natural whole food diet, and what the gastroenterologist had told him contradicted my advice. With a little prodding, I learned that this respected specialist had told the patient to stop eating nuts, seeds, and popcorn because they were probably getting trapped in his diverticula and causing his bouts of diverticulitis. I immediately remembered that I had been suspicious of this theory while in residency, but I didn't argue with my patient. I just told him to give it a try and see how it went. Meanwhile, I made myself a mental note to research as soon as possible.

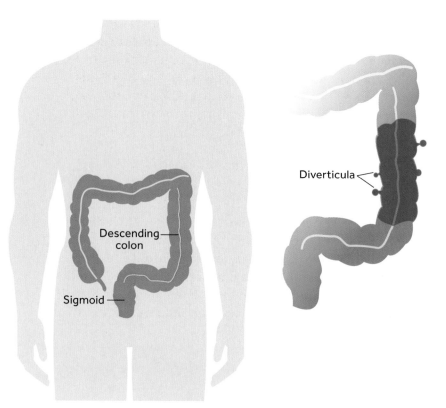

It didn't take me long to find the study I mentioned earlier. There was just one problem. The study had been published in 2008. But even in 2012, the specialist had told my patient to avoid nuts and seeds. I kept rereading the study, thinking that I must be missing something. However, the study showed very clearly that nuts and seeds do not cause flare-ups of diverticulitis. The specialist I had sent my patient to was one of the best in our part of the country. He was very well respected, yet he had told my patient a medical lie—a lie that would not help the patient and actually might harm him. This was *the lie* that made me seriously wonder if there were other lies out there, including lies I had been telling my patients. Did this specialist, whom I greatly respected, not read the medical journals? Did he not research the things he told patients before he shared the information?

I saw this patient again about a month later because he'd had another severe bout of diverticulitis. (I had resisted the urge to call him sooner to tell him of my discovery.) After treating my patient, I gave him a copy of the *JAMA* article. I explained, as respectfully as I could, that the specialist was probably wrong to recommend not eating nuts and seeds. My patient agreed, saying he had avoided all three completely but still had another flare-up. He wanted to know what I thought was causing these flare-ups. I explained what I had read in the article, which said that bouts of diverticulitis were associated with smoking, being overweight, eating red meat, and taking NSAIDs (anti-inflammatory medicines like ibuprofen and naproxen).

My patient was obese, he smoked, and he took ibuprofen almost every day. Armed with this real medical information, he was able to start eating nuts and seeds again (which actually protected him from bouts of diverticulitis), and he was able to refocus his attention on the true causes of his suffering. The specialist hadn't mentioned the patient's weight, smoking habit, or ibuprofen use at all during their visit. The doctor had ordered and performed a colonoscopy (in which a long scope is inserted into the large intestine) and then told the patient to avoid nuts, seeds, and popcorn. That was all he did for my patient.

At first, my patient was skeptical of what I said because I was only his family doctor rather than a specialist. However, he took a copy of the study (I had printed copies to give to patients with diverticulosis) and said he would read it and consider what it had to say. My patient, being a smart man, did just what he promised to do. He returned a few weeks later for my advice on how best to lose some weight and quit smoking. During his visit, he told me that while researching diverticulosis he had discovered hundreds of Internet news articles and blog posts proclaiming the results of the study I had given him. He wanted to know how it was possible that the respected specialist had given him such terrible advice.

I made some excuse for the specialist (doctors are notorious for protecting their own, despite the disastrous consequences of another doctor's ignorance) and steered the conversation back to the patient's diverticulosis. We discussed ways he could control his joint pain aside from taking ibuprofen all the time. Over the next few months, he quit smoking, lost a few pounds, and stopped taking the ibuprofen in favor of getting weekly massage therapy. Now he very rarely (less than once a year) has a flare-up of diverticulitis, even though he eats nuts and seeds every day.

We can, therefore, add diverticulitis to the growing list of things caused by being overweight, smoking, and taking too many pills. We seem to be uncovering a pattern that these three things are dangerous to our long-term health. They won't kill you today, but they will harm you a little each day until the damage builds to the point that it causes a health catastrophe in the future.

You can do an Internet search for diverticulitis and seeds to find hundreds of bloggers and news outlets who know nuts and seeds don't *cause* diverticulitis. Therefore, if your doctor tells you this medical lie, I suggest that you get up and walk out of his office before he finishes his next sentence. He is either unread, lazy, or both, and you can do better for your health. You also could print a copy of the study and mail it to him, or drop off a copy of this book at his office. Maybe he will read it and give better advice to his other patients.

DO AS I DO

I love nuts and seeds and eat some every day. I don't smoke, and I try hard to keep my weight under control. I've never suffered from diverticulitis, but if I ever do, I would still eat nuts and seeds, and you should, too.

HOMEWORK

You can find the JAMA article I mentioned at bit.ly/DivertJAMA. You can read it yourself and print a copy for your doctor. After you read this article, you're going to be at a loss as to why doctors repeat this lie. Please be gentle when you give a copy to your doctor; evidently he can't help perpetuating the myth.

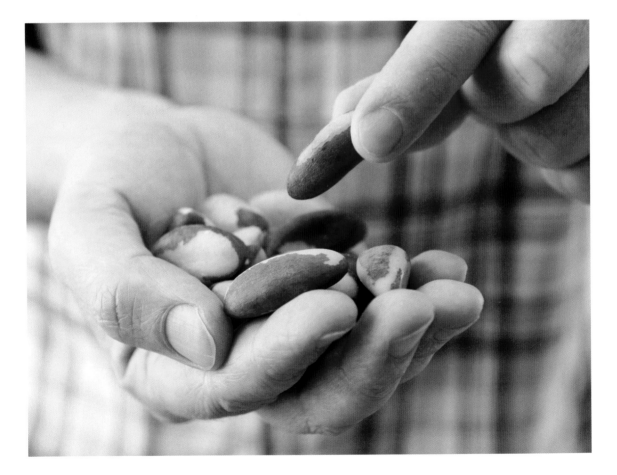

Chapter 10

WILL THIS GIVE MEN PROSTATE CANCER?

"

Formerly, when religion
was strong and science
weak, men mistook magic
for medicine;
now, when science is
strong and religion weak,
men mistake medicine
for magic.

—Thomas Szasz

THE LIE

Giving testosterone to men causes prostate cancer.

WHY YOU SHOULD CARE

As a man ages, his testosterone level drops, which leads to a long list of negative symptoms and suffering. The symptoms can be treated easily with testosterone optimization therapy, which greatly improves a man's quality of life. So if this is a medical lie, we shouldn't be afraid to optimize a man's testosterone. However, if testosterone optimization might cause prostate cancer, then a man shouldn't take the chance of using the therapy.

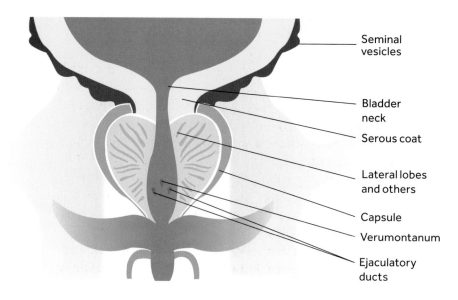

Seminal vesicles

Bladder neck

Serous coat

Lateral lobes and others

Capsule

Verumontanum

Ejaculatory ducts

SUPPORT FOR THE LIE

You'll be surprised when you hear the story of where this lie started and how little meaningful research supports it. It basically comes from one man's opinion, and that opinion wasn't based on any real research. Many other doctors and experts believed the unproven opinion of this one man and have repeated this medical lie for decades.

In the 1940s, Charles B. Huggins, MD, was working with dogs and studying their prostates at the University of Chicago. Dogs and humans are the only animals that have trouble with their prostates becoming enlarged as they age. (Perhaps related to processed food diets? But I digress.) Huggins found that when he castrated the dogs, their prostates shrank. While looking at microscope slides of the dogs' prostates, Huggins noticed areas that looked the same as prostate cancer in humans. When he observed these areas on the slide, he noticed that they were smaller after the dogs had been castrated.

Based on what he had observed in his studies of dogs' prostates, Dr. Huggins did some limited research on humans who had prostate cancer using a lab test that no doctor would use today (acid phosphatase). He concluded that giving a man who has a prostate any testosterone replacement is like throwing gasoline on a fire; the testosterone will increase the risk of developing prostate cancer. He published an article in the very first issue of the journal *Cancer Research* to detail his results. However, he had studied only three men who had received testosterone injections. Furthermore, his report addressed only two of the men, and one of those men had already been castrated. So this medical lie about the connection between testosterone and prostate cancer is based on the results of *one* patient who had already been hormonally manipulated!

Dr. Huggins, although an intelligent expert in his field who was affiliated with a prestigious institution, had based his conclusion on almost no evidence at all. Despite the lack of substantial research to support the theory, a doctor couldn't argue against this medical lie for decades without that doctor being shunned or persecuted by other doctors. Although support for this lie is slowly dying, unthinking or lazy doctors (including urologists) still repeat it.

THE COMMON SENSE

We all start with a testosterone level of zero in the womb, and it goes up from there. We rarely check testosterone levels in healthy children or adults. If, however, a man over forty starts to exhibit symptoms of fatigue, muscle loss, or loss of interest in life, then we check his testosterone levels as part of a complete workup. Male testosterone levels peak between the ages of seventeen and twenty, and then they start to slowly decline. At some point a man's testosterone level gets so low he begins having classic symptoms, such as reduced bone mass, anemia, insomnia, reduced muscle mass, and severe fatigue. When a man's testosterone level gets low enough, he will benefit greatly from having it corrected. Testosterone optimization has been practiced for decades in Europe and California without any increased rate of prostate cancer, but patients have benefited from a definite increase in strength, stamina, and health.

To blindly say that increasing testosterone in a man will increase his risk of prostate cancer is silly. If high testosterone levels were a risk factor for prostate cancer, then male high school seniors would be dying routinely from prostate cancer because their testosterone levels are very high. Think back to your senior year in high school, how many of your classmates had prostate cancer? That's right: not one. But, at that age, a man's testosterone levels are the highest they'll ever be. It's only as a man gets older and his testosterone level drops, or perhaps his testosterone/estrogen ratio drops, that he is at risk for prostate cancer. Prostate cancer is a disease of older men with low testosterone levels. Young men, who have high testosterone levels, never get prostate cancer. Just think about that for a moment. This commonsense fact alone should raise serious doubt about this lie in the average doctor's mind if he is thinking at all.

THE RESEARCH

So, this lie, which has fooled many doctors and caused suffering in many patients, began with research documenting the findings of testosterone therapy on *one* patient. Since then, much research has been done in this area, and virtually all the large, well-done studies show there is no link between optimizing testosterone levels and an increasing risk of prostate cancer.

Each new, properly conducted research study is slowly but surely disproving this medical lie. Researchers are still a little skittish about their research proposals and study conclusions because of past animosity toward this subject, but the tide is inevitably turning to show that testosterone replacement is very good at best and neutral at worst where the incidence of prostate cancer in treated men is concerned. Much more research needs to be done on this topic to find out just how beneficial testosterone optimization is for men.

THE TAKE-HOME

A man feels his best when his testosterone level is in the upper limit of normal. As long as a man's testosterone levels are kept in the upper range of normal, there's no evidence that there are negative risks involved.

Age-Related Decline in Testosterone Levels

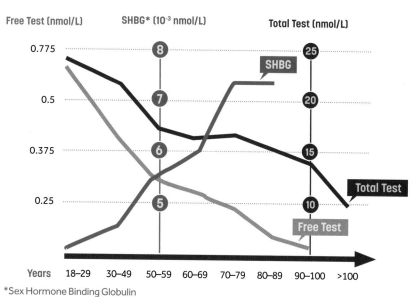

*Sex Hormone Binding Globulin

Many years ago, the average older man's testosterone level was substantially higher than the average older man's level is today. As of now, we're not sure if this was because men previously had better diets, they were more active, or they were exposed to fewer toxic chemicals (or even some other reason). Regardless of the reason today's level is lower than in the past, we need to fix it. I routinely find men in their thirties who have testosterone levels less than 300. (The normal range is 350 to 1,200.) This trend is very concerning because it means that these men, if left untreated, will suffer a slow, painful decline for decades. Doctors need to be optimizing their male patients' testosterone while they search for the environmental and dietary causes of the plummeting average testosterone levels.

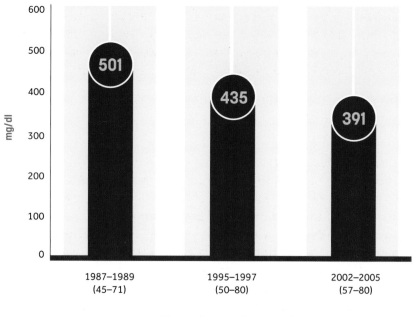

Total Testosterone Concentrations in Men in Massachusetts Male Aging Study

█ Median Total Testosterone

This medical lie is a cautionary tale to all doctors and experts that they should never blindly accept what the prominent leaders in medicine say as absolute truth. Furthermore, patients should never blindly believe what their doctor tells them. Thousands of men have suffered for years and died early, unnecessary deaths because doctors were afraid to check and/or treat their patients' testosterone levels. Men deserve this level of care from their doctor, but they might find they must educate themselves on the subject so they can educate their doctor.

Medical opinion on this subject is currently doing a very slow about-face—at least among doctors who read and think. Experts are now studying the possibility that low testosterone is a cause of prostate cancer, and it seems that keeping a man's testosterone level optimized might protect him from the risk of prostate cancer in addition to preventing many of the other problems of aging. More meaningful research is necessary to clarify this area of medicine, but the current attitude among more progressive doctors is that testosterone optimization is safe, and it's most likely protective against multiple diseases and conditions. If your doctor tells you testosterone optimization is dangerous for you and will increase your risk of prostate cancer, then you have the obvious choice of finding a new doctor, or, if you like your doctor, trying to educate him.

DO AS I DO

I can keep my testosterone levels in the middle to upper range of normal with diet and activity and by avoiding as many toxins as I can. I never eat or drink anything hot from a plastic or Styrofoam container, and I also limit how many canned products I eat. The reason I'm cautious about these situations is because the components in the plastic containers and the can's lining, which contain BPA and/or BPS, are harmful. Many researchers on the subject believe the chemicals in these containers can seep into our food and contribute to lower testosterone levels, along with other problems. The minute I can't maintain a decent testosterone level with diet, exercise, and lifestyle choices, I will work with my doctor to optimize my testosterone level with a bioidentical testosterone replacement.

HOMEWORK

More and more good books and websites are addressing how men can optimize their testosterone levels. I've listed the ones I find most helpful for dispelling myths and giving good, useful information. The more you read, the less afraid you'll be about keeping your testosterone levels in the upper range of normal.

BOOK: *Testosterone for Life* by Abraham Morgentaler, MD (2008)

This Harvard professor tells it like it is. After reading this book, you'll have no fear of optimizing your testosterone level.

BOOK: *The Life Plan* by Jeffry S. Life, MD (2012)

Dr. Life offers great detail about testosterone optimization and other topics older men need to know. He teaches by leading and by setting a great example for other men to follow.

BOOK: *Estrogeneration: How Estrogenetics Are Making You Fat, Sick, and Infertile* by Anthony Jay, PhD (2017)

If you think BPA is the only thing that should worry you about plastics, then this book will really wake you up. Dr. Jay explores all the ways plastics can degrade your health.

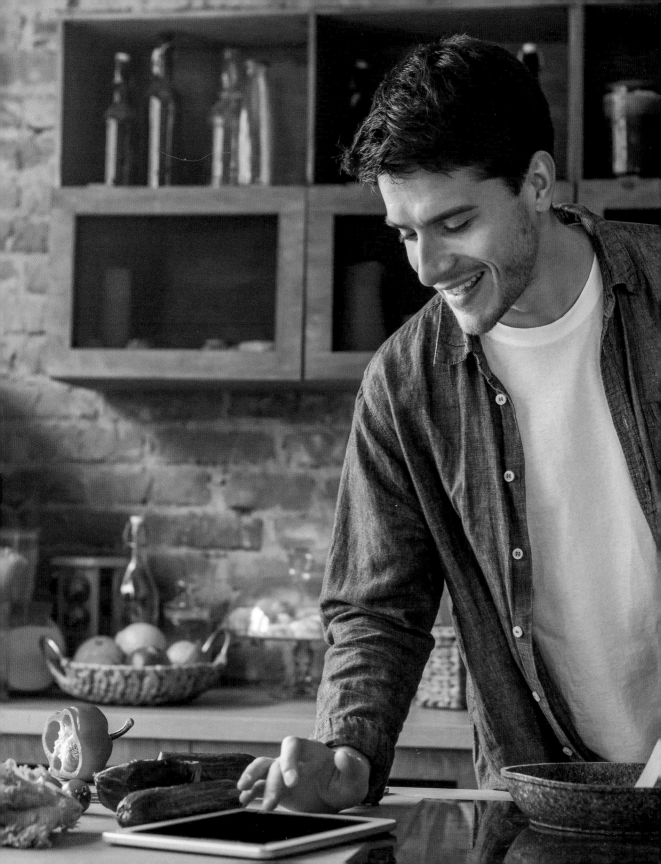

Chapter 11

THERE IS MORE TO WOMEN THAN ESTROGEN

"

Doctors are men who
prescribe medicines of
which they know little,
to cure diseases of which
they know less,
in human beings of which
they know nothing.

—Voltaire

THE LIE

Menopausal women usually don't need progesterone, and they definitely don't need testosterone. If they need anything at all, they need only synthetic estrogen to control hot flushes.

WHY YOU SHOULD CARE

Your hormones, more than anything else in your body, make you who you are. If your hormones are optimal, then so are you. If your hormones are lacking, then so are you. An informed doctor can diagnose and treat low hormone levels with ease. You deserve to feel your best. If optimizing all three female hormones is safe and leads to more enjoyment in life, then a woman should do it. If all that women need to be their best is fake estrogen, then we shouldn't worry about testosterone and progesterone.

SUPPORT FOR THE LIE

Women have unwittingly drawn the short straw as patients for hundreds of years. For example, *hysteria* and *hysterectomy* have the same root, which is from the Greek word for womb *(hustera).* In the past, doctors thought that when a woman acted too hysterical (outside the social norms of the time), it was because the uterus was wandering through her body and making her crazy. The solution was for her to have a hysterectomy (surgical removal of the uterus). No, I'm not kidding. That was the standard of care for medical diagnosis and treatment for many years. The smartest doctors and experts in the country at that time agreed on this diagnosis and treatment plan for thousands of women. (Keep this story in mind when your doctor tells you a medical lie and then says that all the experts say the same thing.)

Therefore, don't be too surprised to hear doctors say silly things such as, "Menopausal women never need any hormone other than estrogen." And by estrogen, they mean synthetic (fake) estrogen. Doctors might also say, "Women don't need testosterone because they don't make it naturally." I've heard licensed, practicing doctors say both of these things. Saying such a thing out loud is embarrassingly ignorant, and treating patients in this manner borders on malpractice. Healthy premenopausal woman *do* make testosterone naturally. Suffice it to say there is little or no meaningful research on either side of this question, as unfair as that is. Historically, doctors and Big Pharma haven't cared enough about menopausal females' comfort and health to thoroughly study this issue except in instances when the goal was to get a new billion-dollar baby (drug) approved by the FDA.

Let me give you an idea of the poor treatment women have gotten from modern medicine when it comes to their hormones by telling you the story of taking testosterone pills. There used to be a testosterone pill on the market for men that would increase their testosterone levels. It was called methyl-testosterone, and it was marketed under several brand names. Although the pill was considered safe initially, it was later determined that taking methylated testosterone by mouth could be toxic for men's livers. The pill was no longer prescribed to men. However, this same methylated testosterone is still readily available for women as part of a combination pill that includes fake estrogen (Estratest)!

Yes, that's right. Either women's livers are magically tougher than men's, or somehow their livers just don't matter as much. Either way, I don't prescribe oral testosterone to either my male or female patients because I believe that, based on the research, it's bad for the liver, no matter who you are. If you're a woman and your doctor has been prescribing this oral testosterone, ask him how it's safe for your liver but not for your husband's or brother's liver. You should also ask him on what research he's basing his decision.

THE COMMON SENSE

According to the feedback from my patients, when women are in their late teens and early twenties, they typically feel the best they will ever feel. Their bodies look and behave how they want them to, and their mood is much more predictable and stable. For women in this age group, the rate of breast and other cancers are extremely low (almost zero). However, if we believe the average doctor's current thinking, women in this age group should have high occurrences of breast cancer and uterine cancer because their hormones are so high.

The doctor uses this same *logic* when he tells a patient who wants to optimize her hormone levels in her forties and later that it will increase her risk of cancer. If it doesn't make sense that high hormone levels increase a woman's cancer risk when she's in her twenties, then it doesn't make sense when she's in her sixties or seventies as long as she uses bioidentical hormones. Big Pharma has produced synthetic estrogens (Premarin, Prempro, and estradiol), and even though they have been proven to increase a woman's risk of cancer, many doctors are still comfortable prescribing them, at least for a few years. However, this same doctor will most likely be very uncomfortable prescribing bioidentical hormones, which should be safe. I recommend that a woman use only bioidentical hormones to optimize her hormone levels.

THE RESEARCH

There is very little meaningful research on women's hormone needs during and after menopause. Researchers did just enough research to show the synthetic estrogens in products like Premarin were sufficiently safe for the FDA to approve the pills. After that, all meaningful research stopped. There are many studies (sponsored by Big Pharma) that demonstrate that one fake estrogen is better than another. However, no studies have been done to compare synthetic estrogens to bioidentical estrogens, although this research should be at the top of the to-do list for doctors in this field.

When it comes to progesterone and testosterone, the story really gets embarrassing. Even now, most doctors tell their patients that progesterone acts only on a woman's uterus; if she doesn't have a uterus, they say she doesn't need progesterone. Apparently we're to assume that the progesterone receptors in a woman's brain were put there to serve no purpose. Doctors view testosterone in much the same way. Most doctors have no idea that a woman needs testosterone to feel, act, and look her best. These doctors will tell you it's unnatural and dangerous to give women testosterone, even though women have testosterone receptors on their hearts and in their brains. Research is severely lacking in this area of hormone optimization, and it should be an embarrassment to doctors who claim expertise in the field of women's health.

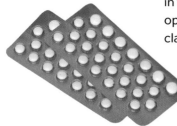

THE TAKE-HOME

There are multiple hormones in the human body, and each one has important effects on multiple organs and systems. It's shameful for a doctor to pretend that all an aging woman needs is either to take a pill for depression or to supplement with a synthetic estrogen to get through a few years of the misery of menopause. In my opinion, it is well within the scope of practice of a good primary care doctor to optimize the hormones of his female patients and help them feel great, stay slimmer, and really enjoy life. Estrogen is certainly very important in this process, but so are testosterone and progesterone.

For a woman to feel her best, she needs to optimize all three hormones. Testosterone is just as important for heart health, energy level, and sense of well-being in a woman as it is in a man. She also needs optimized testosterone levels for good muscle tone, hair, and skin. A woman needs less than one-tenth of the amount of testosterone that a man needs, but without even that small amount, she feels physically exhausted, mentally foggy, and older than her age. Without optimized progesterone levels, anxiety, insomnia, and weight-gain become a menopausal woman's constant companions. Simple lab work before hormone optimization, and regular lab rechecks during therapy, can determine a woman's estrogen, testosterone, and progesterone levels, which makes it possible to keep the levels in the ideal ranges. Optimizing a woman's hormone levels won't change who she is, but it will make her feel like herself again.

If you're a woman who's older than thirty-five, and fatigue, anxiety, insomnia, and/or depression seem to always be plaguing you, ask your doctor to check your hormone levels when he's checking all the other labs that he checks. Ask him which hormones he will check; if he doesn't include testosterone and progesterone, ask him why. If he tells you that a woman doesn't need testosterone—or worse, if he says that it's a male hormone—let the eye-rolling and walking-out begin. (You can also give that doctor a copy of this book as a gift and inscribe it with a strongly worded message.) You deserve to feel your best, and that can happen only if *all* your hormones are optimized. Don't let your doctor's laziness or lack of critical thought keep you from being your best.

DO AS I DO

My wife has her hormone levels checked yearly, and her doctor will begin optimizing her hormones just as soon as her diet and lifestyle no longer keep them in the upper limits of normal. I would be negligent as a husband who is also a doctor if I let her suffer unnecessarily because of falling hormone levels.

HOMEWORK

The mere mention of the fact that women need something other than estrogen as they get older can switch many doctors' minds to the *off* position. Before you go to your next doctor visit, arm yourself with knowledge that will help you open your doctor's eyes or reveal that you need a new doctor. The book I'm suggesting will give you all the knowledge you need to begin your journey back to optimal hormone health. The author is a doctor who's a real advocate of women's health and a leading authority on the real hormone needs of women.

BOOK: *The Secret Female Hormone: How Testosterone Replacement Can Change Your Life* by Kathy C. Maupin, MD (2015)

Dr. Maupin has been an expert in gynecology for decades, and she gives women empowering information about everything their bodies need to be optimal.

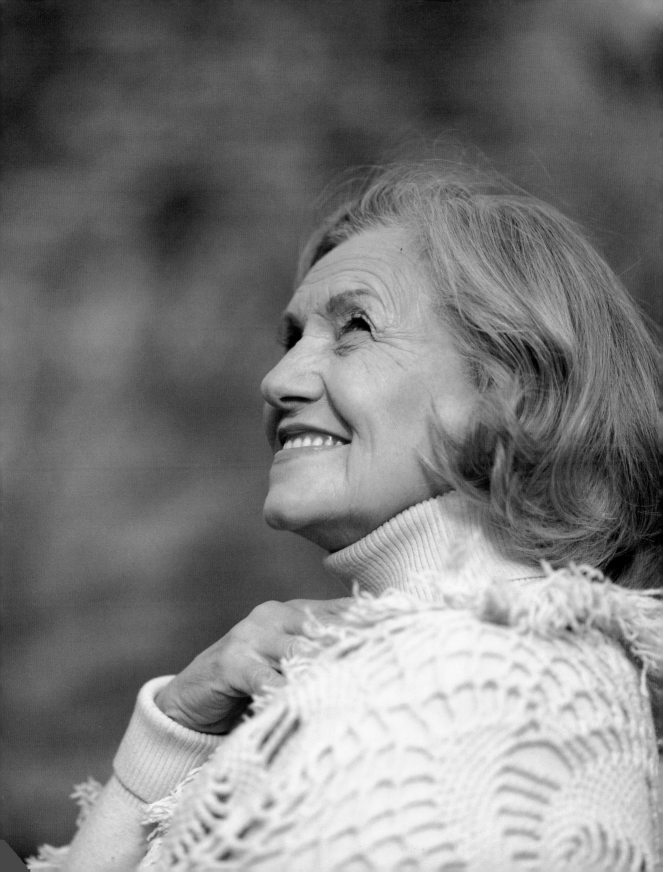

Chapter 12
VIRUSES LAUGH
AT ANTIBIOTICS

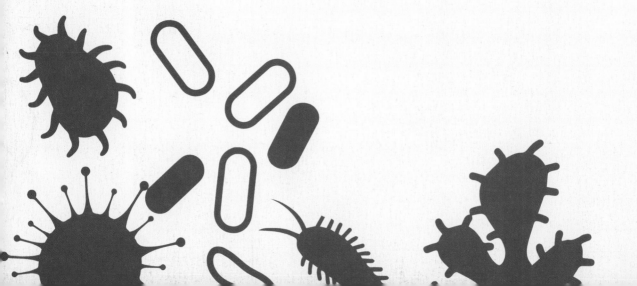

> **"** Drugs are of price value when needed, but they are at best emergency measures of most temporary utility... The more effective they are in the right place, the more harmful in the wrong one.

—Woods Hutchinson

THE LIE

Your runny nose, earache, or cough won't get better unless you take a course of antibiotics. If you take an antibiotic, you will get over your runny nose, earache, or cough more quickly.

WHY YOU SHOULD CARE

Even though we have been trained to think that taking antibiotics is no big deal, in truth it's a very big deal to take a course of antibiotics. The antibiotic can be dangerous to you while you take it, and it also can cause long-term issues with your health. If there are certain types of infections that don't respond to antibiotics, then we shouldn't take the risk of using antibiotics for those infections. For infections that do respond to antibiotics, we should weigh the risks and benefits of taking antibiotics to address them. When we take antibiotics, we always should consider additional steps to minimize other complications of taking the antibiotics.

SUPPORT FOR THE LIE

Since penicillin became known for its lifesaving bacteria-killing properties, humankind has rushed to receive this seemingly miraculous class of medicines. There is no doubt that antibiotics have saved many lives. It's also true that many a life has been taken, or made miserable, by inappropriate antibiotic use. Extensive research shows that antibiotics are effective against certain bacteria, and the research demonstrates the benefits of taking the drugs. Unfortunately, both laziness and the quest for money have led to the gross overuse of antibiotics for infections that aren't responsive to antibiotics or that would have resolved on their own without medicine of any kind. Of course, antibiotics work well under the right circumstances; there's no question about that. The question is why your doctor prescribes them so often when you don't need them and they're not helpful.

For decades, doctors have been telling this medical lie in deed if not in words. Even if your doctor has pamphlets in the waiting room about how colds and other infections are caused by viruses that don't respond to antibiotics, you might still leave his office with a prescription for antibiotics. It's almost as if doctors have been trained by demanding patients to prescribe antibiotics even when they aren't needed.

Compare and Contrast

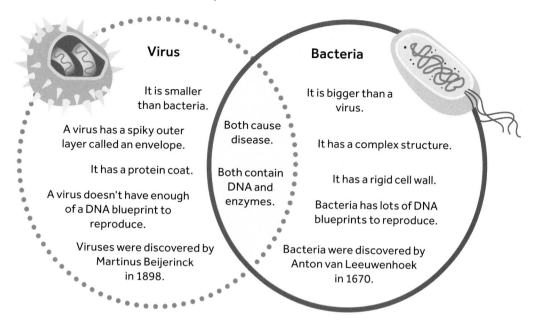

Virus

It is smaller than bacteria.

A virus has a spiky outer layer called an envelope.

It has a protein coat.

A virus doesn't have enough of a DNA blueprint to reproduce.

Viruses were discovered by Martinus Beijerinck in 1898.

Both cause disease.

Both contain DNA and enzymes.

Bacteria

It is bigger than a virus.

It has a complex structure.

It has a rigid cell wall.

Bacteria has lots of DNA blueprints to reproduce.

Bacteria were discovered by Anton van Leeuwenhoek in 1670.

THE COMMON SENSE

Taking any medicine when you don't need it is foolish and possibly dangerous. Medicines, including antibiotics, are powerful and potentially life-threatening tools; you should use them only in the proper amounts and in the proper circumstances. We've all learned since childhood that germs and bacteria are bad, and we should destroy as many of them as we can. We use all kinds of antibacterial products to destroy any bacteria that we come in contact with. Every homemaker's dream of a perfectly clean counter includes a bacterial count of zero.

It turns out the dream of a bacteria-free life is a recent phenomenon. Companies that are trying to sell products for profit are the primary proponents of the concept. We have lived with bacteria, viruses, and fungi—both on us and in us—since the beginning of time. It's true that some of these things are very bad for us, but the vast majority of them range from neutral to beneficial. In your body, bacterial DNA outnumbers your DNA by one hundred to one. Bacteria, like people, can be friends, foes, or neutral entities. The job of doctors is to decide which type of bacteria you have and to use antibiotics only against the dangerous foes.

THE RESEARCH

Research on the effects of bacteria on the human body takes several directions. I can roughly summarize it with the following statements.

- Bacteria do not cause most infections.

- Antibiotics do not work at all on viral infections.

- Viral infections last for a few days (three to fourteen) and then go away.

- Some bacteria can make us very sick or even kill us.

- Some bacteria are beneficial to us.

- Antibiotics kill many bacteria, both bad and good.

- Antibiotics can't kill some bacteria.

- Overuse of antibiotics can lead to resistant bacteria.

- Killing good bacteria can have negative health consequences.

- Taking antibiotics can lead to weight gain.

- Wise use of antibiotics often means *not* using them.

I know this list may seem complicated, but the subject of bacteria and antibiotic use is complicated and clouded. All the latest research, as well as expert opinion, seems to be trending in the right direction: We should use antibiotics only in certain situations, we should use them only for a limited time, and we should avoid them at all costs in every other situation.

THE TAKE-HOME

We have lived in the muck and mud for most of our time on this planet. Being dirty was the rule rather than the exception for most of our existence as a species. Our immune system has been learning from, and even working with, these bacteria for eons. You have so many bacteria inside of you right now that it's valid to wonder whether the bacteria belong to you, or you belong to them. Only a very few bacteria in very few situations are dangerous; those are the bacteria that we should treat with antibiotics.

Any time you take antibiotics for a cold or other viral illness, two things occur:

- The antibiotic has no effect on the cause of your illness or on the number of days you will be sick.

- The antibiotics kill billions of beneficial bacteria in your gut and other places in and on your body. That bacterial slaughter can have a negative effect on your health in many ways.

As we learn more about beneficial bacteria, we're finding that they do everything from protecting our skin from the environment to helping us remain slimmer to keeping us from developing autoimmune diseases.

It's likely that bacteria serve us in hundreds of ways we don't fully understand. When we consider how much we don't know about bacteria, it quickly becomes obvious that we should be exceptionally careful about doing anything that might damage these herds of good and gentle bacteria. Here's an analogy about the effects of taking an antibiotic for every little infection: Imagine you're a farmer who has a fire-ant nest in your pasture. Because the fire ants (a virus) are stinging you and your cows, you hire an expert (a doctor) to get rid of them, and the expert's treatment is to set off a huge cluster bomb (prescribe an antibiotic) in your pasture (your body). When the smoke clears, you would be excited to see that all the fire ants on your farm had been destroyed, but you'd be devastated to see that the expert had also killed all your cattle as well. To add insult to injury, the expert's bomb also knocked over your barn. You don't have to be a wise farmer to know that the cluster bomb is a very bad strategy.

Some doctors are quick to blame their patients for the overuse of antibiotics. However, the truth is that the problem is not with antibiotic overuse; the problem is in the overprescribing of

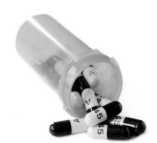

antibiotics. When a worried parent brings a sick child to the doctor for care, it is not the parent's fault if the doctor gives in to the demands for an antibiotic. The parent is only trying to make sure the child's health improves. We wouldn't say that it's the diabetic patient's fault if the doctor prescribes too much insulin, right? We also wouldn't say that it's the drug-addicted patient's fault if the doctor prescribes more narcotics, right? And it isn't the parent's fault if the doctor prescribes the child antibiotics just because the parent has demanded them. The doctor should know when antibiotics are truly called for and refuse to prescribe them whenever they aren't necessary. In my opinion, this is one area where state medical boards should be much more active in policing medical professionals by sanctioning and fining doctors who overprescribe antibiotics.

The best way to be sure your doctor doesn't give you an antibiotic for a viral infection is to not go to the doctor when you have a runny nose, scratchy throat, and a cough. Viruses always cause these symptoms, and there is no magic pill that makes them go away one second sooner than they would without the pill. Your doctor wants badly to help you and for you to see him as being good at what he does. When you see him for a problem he can't help you with, you kick his human nature, which I talk about in Chapter 2, into gear. His inclination is probably to do something rather than nothing, even if the something leads to negative long-term consequences. Doing nothing is very difficult for most doctors to do, even though doing nothing might be the exact treatment you need at the time.

An infection or an illness is often not caused by a bacterial villain; it's caused by a bacterial imbalance that allowed a viral infection to happen. As we learn more about this subject, we're finding that a better strategy than killing bacteria is to put even more bacteria (good bacteria) into your system. Probiotics are becoming very popular and, although we still have much to learn about the amounts and varieties needed for different conditions, it's becoming obvious that using probiotics is a much more effective strategy than setting off an antibiotic cluster bomb in your body.

You should take a course of antibiotics only if it is certain that a bacterial infection is causing your illness, if the illness probably won't go away on its own, and if the illness caused by the bacterial infection presents a risk of significant danger to you. If you go to your doctor with a runny nose, cough, and low-grade fever, you do not need antibiotics. If your doctor prescribes antibiotics for you, he is hurting your health, not helping it. Only rarely in your life will you need well-chosen, carefully administered antibiotics. If your doctor seems to give you antibiotics almost every time you make an office visit, ask him why it's his go-to course of action and request a copy of the research that backs up his prescriptions.

DO AS I DO

I haven't taken antibiotics in years. Fortunately, I rarely suffer from infections of any kind, but when I do have a viral infection, antibiotics are the last thing on my mind. Probiotics have a daily place in my supplement regimen, and I find this prevents most infections that other people suffer. Only if I had some specific severe bacterial infections would I even consider taking an antibiotic.

HOMEWORK

I'm so glad the table is finally turning on this issue. More and more doctors and experts are realizing antibiotics are dangerous tools that they should use only in specific situations. The following two books describe in elegant detail just how important it is to have the right bacteria. After reading these books, you will protect and nourish your bacteria rather than cluster-bombing them.

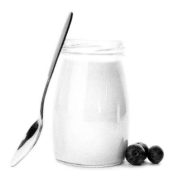

BOOK: *10% Human: How Your Body's Microbes Hold the Key to Health and Happiness* by Alanna Collen, PhD (2016)

This brilliant book explains, in interesting detail, how many bacteria you contain, all the good things they do for you, and why it's a bad idea to be mean to them. This book is a must-read for all doctors and patients.

BOOK: *Missing Microbes: How the Overuse of Antibiotics Is Fueling Our Modern Plagues* by Martin J. Blaser, MD (2015)

This book is a very informative work that explains the damage that we have done and all the negative health consequences we experience from overusing antibiotics.

Chapter 13
SALT OF THE EARTH

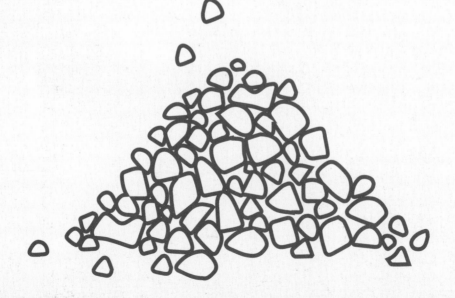

**We are in the age of M.D.,
medical darkness,
which seeks legislative
protection from the light.**

—James Lendall Basford

THE LIE

Eating salt increases your risk of having high blood pressure, which increases your risk for heart attack and stroke. You should eat a low-salt diet as much as possible to prevent heart disease.

WHY YOU SHOULD CARE

Obviously, you would like to avoid having a heart attack. You would also like to enjoy good-tasting food. The worst possible outcome of this situation would be to endure years of a bland, salt-free Food Pyramid diet and then still have an early heart attack. If eating salt truly does increase heart attack and stroke risk, then we should avoid salt and eat bland foods. If eating salt is safe, then we can relax and salt our food to taste. When you're busy worrying about something that doesn't increase your risk of heart attack, like salt, then you will not be focusing on things that do increase your chances of a heart attack (such as insulin resistance, chronic inflammation, obesity, and alcohol abuse).

SUPPORT FOR THE LIE

The educated opinion of nearly every scientist and doctor in the world is that eating less salt leads to lower blood pressure, thus decreasing your chances of suffering from an early heart attack. For some reason, this medical lie caught on so strongly that, even though there was no real evidence to support it, and little money to be made from it, almost every doctor piled on the bandwagon to bad-mouth salt. Hundreds of articles in every publication, from the most scientific journal to the lowliest gossip rag, supported the idea that eating salt increases your blood pressure and your chances of having a heart attack. However, if you look closely at the scientific literature, even at articles that supposedly proved the salt-hypertension link, it's clear the conclusions were stretched to the limits of believability. Time and again, meaningful research has failed to show any link between enjoying salt with your meals and increased blood pressure (or increased heart attack risk).

THE COMMON SENSE

For all our existence on this planet we have loved salt and have eaten as much as we wanted or could find. All mammals crave salt and will travel impressive distances to enjoy it. A desire so hardwired into all mammals usually means that we need that substance to survive. Farmers put huge blocks of salt in their barns because the cows love to lick it. The salt is good for cows—not bad. In actuality, it's very difficult for a normal cow, or person, to eat too much salt. A person with healthy kidneys can easily urinate away excess salt. If you have kidney disease, then you should discuss your salt intake with your doctor.

THE RESEARCH

Hundreds of studies have been done on both sides of this argument, but three large, well-done studies leave little doubt about this lie:

- A 2003 Cochran review of fifty-seven trials stated, "There is little evidence for long-term benefit from reducing salt intake."

- In 2006, The American Journal of Medicine recorded the salt intake of more than 70 million Americans and compared it to their risk of dying from heart disease over a fourteen-year period. What did the study find? The more sodium people ate, the less likely they were to die from heart disease. (Yep, you read that right).

- The American Journal of Hypertension included a study of more than 8,000 participants. The results reflected that salt had virtually no impact on blood pressure.

So with all this research proving that decreasing salt intake gives no protection from increasing blood pressure or heart attack, why do doctors still tell this medical lie? I honestly have no idea.

THE TAKE-HOME

This medical lie is a fine example of well-meaning experts who believe something, and they try to *help* humankind by pushing that belief onto everyone else. The ideas and research the experts based their assumptions on were flawed; thus, the conclusions were inaccurate. Because of this, doctors give misguided advice to millions of patients. These patients have had to suffer from bland low-sodium diets, which tasted awful, and (according to the one study) actually increased their odds of having a heart attack.

When the experts first published their beliefs about high salt intake, the regulatory bodies (FDA, USDA, AHA, AMA) picked up this lie and ran with it, spreading it even farther than the original research would have traveled. Then every doctor told his patients the lie because he believed he was doing them a favor. Finally, your mom, your brother, and your next-door neighbor were yelling at you every time you picked up the salt shaker. Eventually, as the decades pass, this medical lie will slip into oblivion. Doctors will stop saying it, and, later still, so will everyone else.

Unless you have poor kidney function or significant heart failure, you're free to relax your fears and eat salt to taste on all your food. Humans with healthy kidneys and adequate water intake can eat as much salt as they want. Salt will not hurt them or elevate their blood pressure. They will excrete the extra salt with each full bladder of urine they release.

The human body has very strict mechanisms for keeping the proper amounts of sodium, chloride, and other electrolytes in salt in the bloodstream and tissues. Thinking that eating a little extra salt on your dinner will somehow screw up these mechanisms is silly. Unprocessed sea salt is a little better for you than processed table salt. However, that just means that the processed table salt is less good than the sea salt, but it's not truly bad. The best choice for salt, though, is unprocessed pink or gray sea salt because most of us are deficient in some mineral or another, and the sea salts can help boost these deficiencies. With sea salt, you get all the flavor you want and the multiple minerals your body needs.

If you see your doctor and he tells you to reduce your sodium or salt intake to lower your blood pressure or address some other health issue, please try to take it easy on him. He's repeating a medical lie that's only now starting to die slowly. Many good doctors haven't done the reading they need to be able to see past the lie. You can ask a respectful question about what research he is basing his advice on; that might be enough to motivate him to put on his reading glasses and begin getting up to date. This lie is another great example of how patients can begin to take control of their health, research as deeply as they want into the subject, and begin to take pride in their knowledge and their improving health. Addressing this medical lie with your doctor can be the beginning of a much stronger partnership between the two of you. Either he will do his reading and become a better doctor, or he will be rude to you, which gives you an opportunity to find a new doctor.

DO AS I DO

We always have salt on our table and in our kitchen. We use salt in virtually every dish we prepare. I've never liked the taste of too much salt, but I have no fear of using it. We use unprocessed Himalayan sea salt that we grind ourselves, and we put it in everything. Even if I do develop a blood pressure problem later in life, I will continue to use my sea salt without fear.

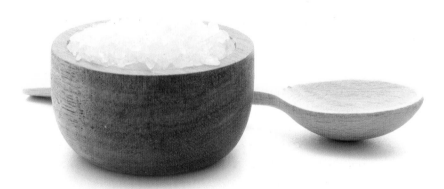

HOMEWORK

Salt is necessary for optimized human health, but you will probably need some knowledge bullets in your gun when you attack your doctor with this idea. I'm suggesting two great books and a magazine article that describe all the benefits of eating good salt. The magazine article also includes all the dumb things that experts and government agencies have said and done about salt.

BOOK: *The Salt Fix* by James DiNicolantonio, PhD (2017)

Dr. DiNicolantonio dives deep into the science to show that salt is a vital, healthy substance for humans, and it can even enhance physical performance.

BOOK: *Salt Your Way to Health* by David Brownstein, MD (2006)

Dr. Brownstein has been bucking the system for decades. This book is full of great ideas and great information about salt and its health benefits.

MAGAZINE ARTICLE: "It's Time to End the War on Salt" by Melinda Wenner Moyer in *Scientific American* (July 2011)

Ms. Moyer gives a great summary of the history of making salt a health no-no and explains how state and federal health experts have bungled this issue. Some of the decisions made at the federal level are embarrassing, to say the least.

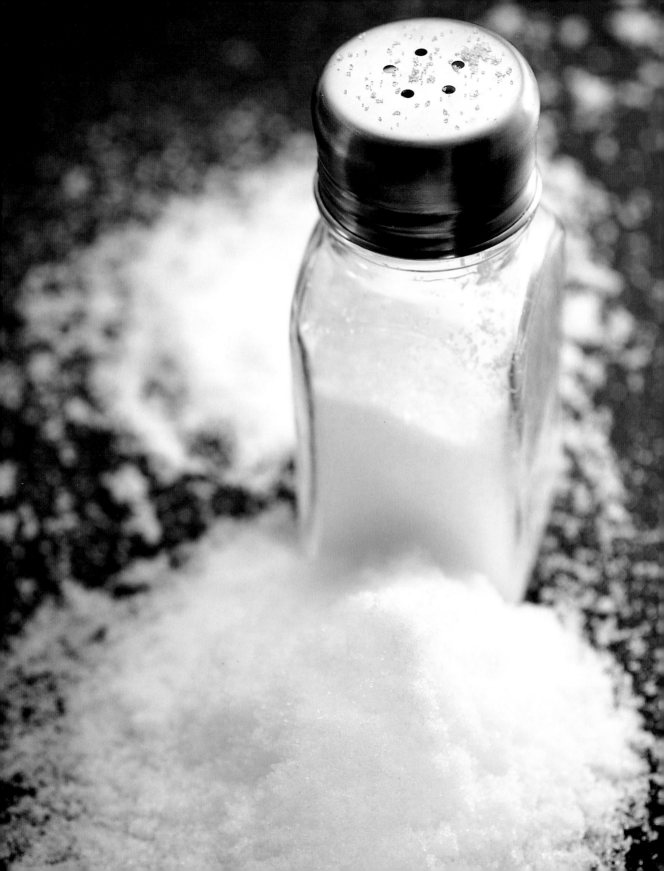

Chapter 14

ALL CALORIES ARE NOT CREATED EQUAL

"

What some call health, if purchased by perpetual anxiety about diet, isn't much better than tedious disease.

—George Dennison Prentice

"

THE LIE

A calorie is a calorie; whether the source is birthday cake or broccoli. You can eat whatever you want as long as you limit your total calorie intake. You will be slender and healthy by counting calories because all calories are the same. If you want to lose weight, then you should burn more calories than you eat.

WHY YOU SHOULD CARE

If this medical lie were true, it would let you think of junk food and special treats the same way you think of nourishing food. Birthday cake is not a nourishing food, but if you consider the calories in it to have the same effect on your body as the calories in broccoli, then the cake is a valid food choice. According to this lie, your only concern is that you don't go over your total calorie limit each day.

If this lie is true, then you can eat whatever you want as long as you watch your total calorie count. If the total calorie count of the foods you eat is not important, then you should be careful to eat real, whole foods daily and to enjoy treats only occasionally. Good health is built on the foundation of a good diet. We must know what really matters and what things we should spend our money and our effort on if we want to have a strong mind and a healthy body.

SUPPORT FOR THE LIE

Most doctors and magazine articles imply that a calorie from one food is the same as a calorie from any other food. Nutrition experts often tell us that a calorie of cake is no different than a calorie of spinach. Scientists and a few doctors stopped repeating this lie years ago because they had crunched the numbers from large research studies and had shown this belief to be false and not worthy of being repeated. I can find very few medical studies that specifically examine this lie. It is repeated mainly as unsupported, expert opinion. Lazy doctors and concerned family members are now the main repeaters of this medical lie, but it is still out there causing people to make dietary mistakes.

You may have read or heard that fat has more calories per gram than protein or carbohydrates. This statement is true if you burn your food in a little furnace (like the one in the illustration below), but it makes absolutely no difference as far as your health and weight-loss goals are concerned. Your digestive system breaks down your food biochemically; it doesn't burn your food as a furnace would. Lazy doctors repeat this type of "fact" because they don't know any better and don't make an effort to learn the truth. Many a well-intentioned doctor has instructed their patients that the key to weight loss is to burn more calories than they eat. The doctors tell the patients that a daily *calorie deficit* will lead to weight loss.

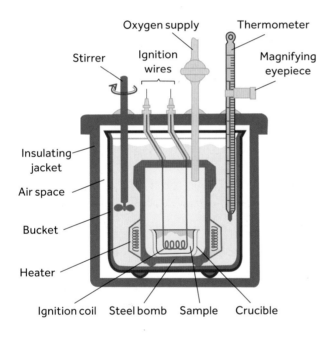

THE COMMON SENSE

The way that most of us have learned the calorie paradigm, it would seem to make sense that a calorie is a calorie, no matter what the food source. Scientists came up with the whole concept of a food calorie by burning small amounts of different foods in a little furnace. They measured the escaping heat to determine the calories in the food. The number of calories shown beside a given food has absolutely nothing to do with how the human body metabolizes the food; it tells you only how many calories of heat-energy were created by burning the food in that little furnace. We don't burn the food we eat; we *digest* it. Common sense really doesn't apply to this lie because the lie itself is nonsensical; we were taught a silly way of describing the *energy* contained in different foods.

The biochemistry used by the human body is extremely complicated. The analogy that we burn the food we eat is a bad one that misleads our thinking on the subject. Don't let a doctor or nutritionist tell you they know everything there is to know about how the body uses our food and stores energy; it just isn't true. The calorie was invented as a way for scientists to talk about the heat energy in food, but it has nothing to do with how healthy a given food is or whether that food will cause you to gain or lose weight.

THE RESEARCH

There is minimal research that supports this lie. Research has been done to determine the calorie count of virtually every food on the planet. However, there is little research showing that the human body cares about the calorie-count of your food, or agrees with the laboratory count of calories in a food or beverage.

No meaningful research has ever shown that a calorie of cake is the same, from a health and obesity standpoint, as a calorie of bacon or a calorie of artichoke. The "fact" that all calories are equivalent was accepted by the medical and nutrition communities as self-evident, and this medical lie became the basis for all nutritional advice.

A 2012 article in *JAMA* definitively laid this medical lie to rest. The study analyzed three groups of patients who all ate the same total number of calories daily. One group ate a high-carbohydrate diet, one group ate a high-protein diet, and one group ate a high-fat diet. Which group do you think lost the most weight? Based on what you've learned your whole life, you probably didn't choose the high-fat diet participants, but that group lost more weight than either of the other two groups. Your doctor should have read this article and should know not to be wasting your time talking about counting calories and eating a low-fat diet.

THE TAKE-HOME

Doctors are very busy, and most of them don't understand that being very educated about nutrition is much more important for their patients' health than knowing about the newest pill or shot from Big Pharma. Doctors don't want to be nutritionists; they want to be experts on drugs and medical procedures. Very few doctors seem to realize that most prescription drugs and medical procedures wouldn't be necessary if patients were educated and encouraged to follow a proper diet. I often wonder what the average doctor's answer would be if a patient asked, "Do you think type 2 diabetes is curable?" or "How important do you think nutrition is in preventing heart attack, stroke, and cancer?" I'm afraid the most likely answers would be "No," and "Somewhat important, but not as important as these medications you can take." A good primary care doctor should be an expert on the latest nutritional research and be able to educate his patients about ways to eat to reach and maintain a healthy weight. He should also apply his advice to himself and set a good example for his patients.

A good way to look at this issue is to examine medical advice and obesity rates over the last thirty years. During this time, people have repeated the advice that one calorie is no worse than any other calorie, but the general trend of the population has been to gain weight. The increased obesity of the population doesn't support the idea that a calorie from broccoli is no better than a calorie from a cookie. Counting calories is a complete waste of time. It squanders your valuable energy and motivation by keeping you busy doing something that doesn't help with weight loss, thus almost guaranteeing you will fail.

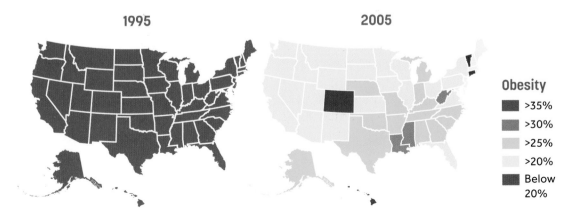

1995 2005

Obesity
- >35%
- >30%
- >25%
- >20%
- Below 20%

2017

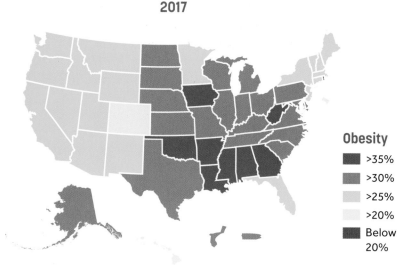

Obesity
- >35%
- >30%
- >25%
- >20%
- Below 20%

When the average person becomes motivated to lose weight and get healthier, they usually start counting calories with gusto. They will continue for a month or two, but after seeing minimal results, they will get discouraged and slowly stop trying. (Sound familiar?) Sometimes this poor patient's doctor will make the person feel guilty for giving up, which is outrageous because this very same doctor is the person who gave the patient the bad advice that led to the failure. It's not fair for the patient to be made to feel guilty for giving up on a stupid concept that doesn't work in the first place! If a large part of your current *diet* plan consists of counting and keeping up with calories, then you will ultimately fail. Counting calories doesn't help and doesn't work if your goal is long-term permanent weight loss and improved health. You need to start doing research about how humans should eat and what helps them attain an ideal body weight.

When you're ready and motivated to lose extra weight, you want your effort to produce maximum weight loss. You don't want to put a lot of effort toward this goal to lose a few pounds before gaining them right back. You want to do what will give results immediately and will work permanently. If your doctor tells you the key to losing weight is to cut back on calories and exercise more, please try to contain your anger. Perhaps he has recently been released from solitary confinement where he was not allowed to read any medical journals for the last few years. You might be able to help him by pointing out an article or two that would bring him up to speed.

Tell your doctor that you're going to eat real, whole foods, and you're going to eat them until you're full. You can explain that a calorie of cake is not equal to a calorie of blueberry, so you plan to avoid the former and enjoy the latter. Please don't waste one second of your time, or one calorie of your effort, worrying about calories. They are irrelevant, and your doctor should know that by now. Weight gain is caused by eating the wrong foods and screwing up your insulin metabolism—not by eating too many calories.

DO AS I DO

Eating large amounts of food-products, which were labeled with a long list of strange ingredients, used to be my usual diet plan. After realizing I was a fat-assed, grouchy, fatigued, heartburn-suffering, runny-nosed doctor who shouldn't be giving anyone health or nutrition advice, I changed all that. Now I rarely eat anything that has more than one ingredient. The ingredients in broccoli are—well, *broccoli*. In our house, eating real, whole foods is the rule rather than the exception. The human body and digestive system knows perfectly well what to do with whole foods. It gets confused by foods that come in cardboard boxes and are made with weird ingredients. Your body tends to put those foods directly on your belly or your butt as fat.

HOMEWORK

The *all calories are equal* lie is so stupid that I'm done talking about it. You need to do some homework on what your body *needs* and how it uses the food you eat. I'm suggesting four great books on this subject. The first three titles are the books that introduced me to this topic, and they changed how I think of human nutrition and how I practice medicine. After you've read these three, you will be smarter than 95 percent of the doctors in the world when it comes to human nutrition.

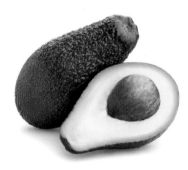

BOOK: *The New Primal Blueprint: Reprogram Your Genes for Effortless Weight Loss, Vibrant Health, and Boundless Energy* by Mark Sisson (2016)

This book really describes the entire lifestyle you need to look (muscular and fit) and feel (happy and energetic) like a hunter-gatherer. (The copy I initially read was an earlier edition.)

BOOK: *The Paleo Diet: Lose Weight and Get Healthy by Eating the Foods You Were Designed to Eat* by Loren Cordain, PhD (2010)

This is one of the best books I've ever read about human health and nutrition. This author grabbed modern nutrition science by the hair and slapped it silly. Slowly but surely, doctors and experts are waking up to the truth of human nutrition.

BOOK: *Dr. Atkins' Diet Revolution: The High Calorie Way to Stay Thin Forever* by Robert Atkins, MD (1972)

I can't even imagine the cold shoulders and stern looks Dr. Atkins must have endured when he initially promoted his book. He was a doctor who thought outside of his box, and he should be knighted or sainted for shifting the paradigm as much as he did . He was a true revolutionary, rest his soul.

BOOK: *Good Calories, Bad Calories: Fats, Carbs, and the Controversial Science of Diet and Health* by Gary Taubes (2008)

The book that first revealed the truth about calories and weight loss that has been known for decades but forgotten by most doctors.

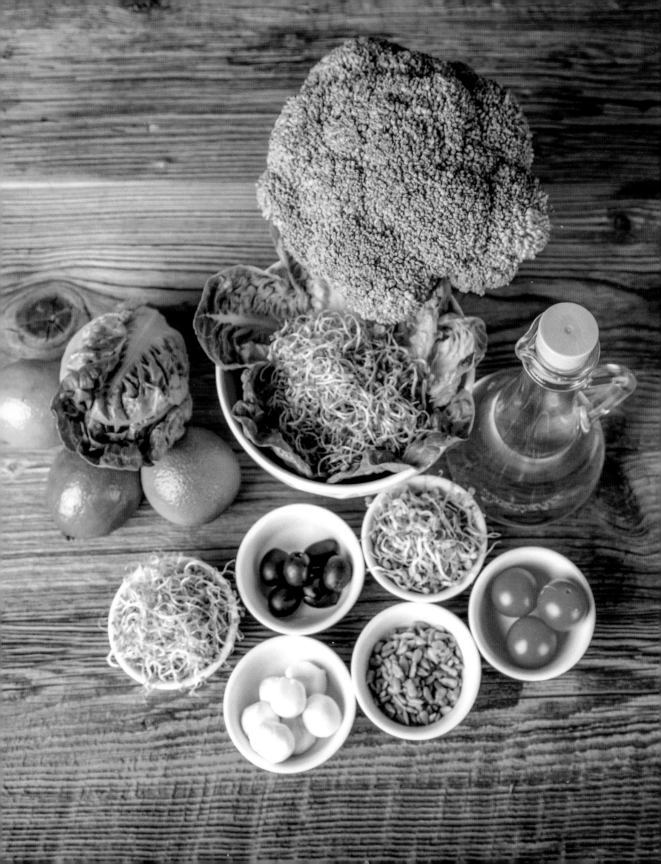

Chapter 15

DOES TOO MUCH CALCIUM CAUSE KIDNEY STONES?

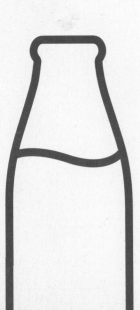

**The art of medicine
consists in amusing the
patient while nature cures
the disease.**

—Voltaire

THE LIE

Eating or drinking too much calcium can lead to kidney stones. Also, if you've had a kidney stone, you should decrease your calcium intake so you don't get another.

WHY YOU SHOULD CARE

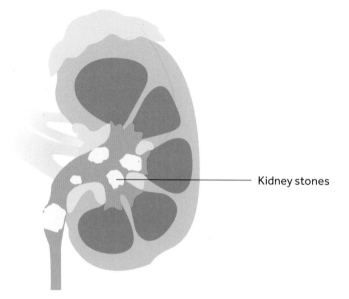

Kidney stones

Large kidney stones are, without doubt, one of the most painful things the human body can experience. Any time a woman describes a pain as worse than childbirth, you better bet you don't want to experience it. I've had multiple women over the years tell me their kidney stones were much more painful than the worst of their labor pains. As a man, all I can do with this information is place the pain at about twenty-five on a ten-point scale and pray I never experience it. No woman has ever described any other pain to me using the childbirth analogy, even when she's had multiple broken bones. So, if high-calcium foods increase your risk of kidney stones, then maybe you should cut down on eating them. But if high-calcium foods don't increase your kidney stone risk, then you can enjoy them as much as you want.

SUPPORT FOR THE LIE

Many people on the street and some doctors will repeat this medical lie as truth. There is absolutely no research showing that high-calcium foods in your diet increase your risk of a kidney stone. There is some mediocre research showing a possible relationship between taking large doses of calcium supplements and developing kidney stones, but the jury is out on this theory until someone performs a meaningful study.

THE COMMON SENSE

Because most kidney stones consist of mostly of calcium, it seems to make sense that eating too much calcium might increase your chances of having a kidney stone. Calcium is vital to building bone and hundreds of other bodily functions, so it stands to reason that you should make sure you get plenty of it. Calcium levels in the blood and urine are tightly controlled by the body's mechanisms. Calcium metabolism is too complicated to be boiled down to a summary as simple as "eating too much will cause your body to produce stones that result in the worst pain known to humans."

THE RESEARCH

No research has ever shown that high levels of calcium in your food and drink increases your risk of a kidney stone. Also, no study has ever shown that those who have had one kidney stone can decrease the risk of having another stone in the future by lowering their calcium intake. A study presented at the ninety-fourth meeting of The Endocrine Society showed a possible link between taking a calcium supplement (pill) and increasing risk of kidney stones, but the evidence was far from convincing.

THE TAKE-HOME

Calcium in your diet does not cause kidney stones. If you have a kidney stone at some point, it does not mean that you should avoid foods that are naturally high in calcium. You can decrease your risk of having a stone, but you can't do it by avoiding calcium in your diet.

For a few years, it was very popular, especially for women, to take a calcium supplement. Although this was probably unnecessary and probably didn't increase their bone strength, we didn't see a sudden uptick in kidney stones in women. The nutrient in which most women are deficient and that most likely will increase bone strength (and help the body's biochemistry in hundreds of ways) is vitamin D3.

Most people get enough calcium in a healthy diet, but it is almost impossible to get enough vitamin D3 in a modern diet. We are told to hide from the sun because too much sun causes cancer, but without exposure to the sun, you're not getting vitamin D the way nature intended. Therefore, most people have to take a vitamin D3 supplement daily. Don't worry about too much calcium in your diet causing kidney stones, but do ask your doctor to order a Vitamin D-25 level for you. Checking your vitamin D level is important.

If your doctor tells you to decrease your calcium intake to keep you from making kidney stones, you should respectfully tell him you would like a copy of the research upon which he's basing his advice. This request will most likely fluster him and give you the perfect opportunity to start working on an improved partnership with him.

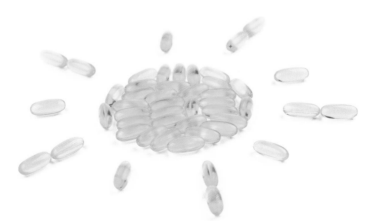

DO AS I DO

I've never had a kidney stone, and I want to keep it that way. Eating a natural whole food diet gives me plenty of calcium (from kale, sardines, broccoli, okra, and almonds). Drinking milk isn't necessary. I also plan to take a vitamin D3 supplement daily as needed until I've saved enough money to move to Key West, where I'll produce plenty of vitamin D from sun exposure, as nature intended.

HOMEWORK

Because the real problem isn't about getting enough or too much calcium, you should do homework about vitamin D instead of reading about calcium. I'm suggesting a web page that will make you an expert on vitamin D, which is a very important nutrient most of us don't get enough of.

WEBSITE: *Vitamin D Resource Page* The Vitamin D Council

The Vitamin D Council has great information about vitamin D at http://bit.ly/VitDFAQ.XBPRRGhKiUk.

Chapter 16
YOUR TSH IS NORMAL, SO YOUR THYROID IS FINE

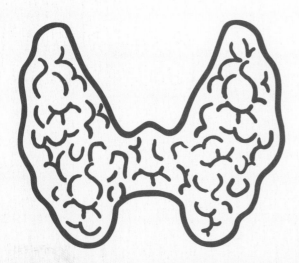

"

It is easy to get a thousand prescriptions but hard to get one single remedy.

—Chinese proverb

"

THE LIE

TSH (thyrotropin stimulating hormone) is all you need to have checked to find out whether your thyroid is functioning normally. If TSH is within normal limits, then your thyroid gland is fine, and your symptoms are all in your head.

WHY YOU SHOULD CARE

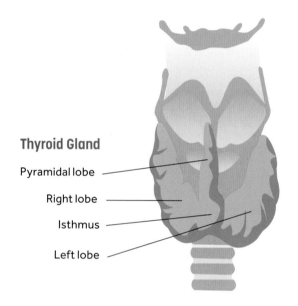

Thyroid Gland

Pyramidal lobe

Right lobe

Isthmus

Left lobe

The thyroid gland and the hormones it produces affect virtually every biochemical reaction in your body. If your thyroid doesn't function properly, the result is fatigue, weight-gain, memory-loss, disease, and even early death. If the TSH test is the only lab test that needs to be checked to assess thyroid health, then so be it. If, however, a full panel of thyroid lab work and the patient's symptoms and signs need to be considered before the doctor makes a diagnosis, then let's make sure to check all of it.

SUPPORT FOR THE LIE

It is the opinion of almost every thyroid specialist (endocrinologist) that if your TSH level is within normal limits, then your thyroid is fine. Recommendations from endocrine societies recommend the TSH test as the only test needed to screen the thyroid gland. All doctors were, and still are, taught this lie in medical school and residency, and they haven't thought much about it since. The TSH test is quick and easy to perform, and the results appear to be undeniable black and white. Very few doctors have any doubt in using the TSH test for diagnosing thyroid disease.

THE COMMON SENSE

Given that the thyroid is known the world over as the master gland of the human body, it would seem that proper diagnosis and treatment of thyroid conditions is vital to long-term health and happiness. Way back in the 1970s, the TSH level became the standard way to test the thyroid. For some reason, doctors (even so-called thyroid specialists) want to bet your thyroid health on this forty-year-old test.

TSH is not even a thyroid hormone; it's a hormone produced by the anterior pituitary gland in the brain. The pituitary produces TSH as the way of telling the thyroid gland to produce more thyroid hormone. When the thyroid hormone level circulating in the blood is at the proper level, it feeds back to the pituitary gland, telling it to stop producing TSH. There are multiple places in this feedback loop where something can go wrong but remain completely undetected in the lab work if your doctor checks only your TSH level.

An article by Colin M. Dayan, FRCP, in the 2001 *Lancet* discussed this potential problem and suggested that at least TSH, FT3, and FT4 should be checked to minimize the chances of overlooking hidden disease. FT3 is free T3, the active form of thyroid hormone that circulates in the blood, and FT4 is free T4, the storage form of circulating thyroid hormone. Even though this doctor told the medical world via a respected medical journal that checking just the TSH was not enough, hard-headed doctors kept right on checking only the TSH.

THE RESEARCH

Research supporting this lie is tenuous at best. When the TSH test became available, doctors were excited about having a fast and easy thyroid test. They basically forgot how to use their critical judgment and physical examination skills where the signs and symptoms of thyroid disease are concerned. They started to blindly trust this one test. Authors of research papers often initially imply that the TSH is all that needs to be checked, but then they waffle later in the article by mentioning something like "the TSH test's weaknesses should be kept in mind." Many doctors have stopped reading before they get to the second part. Therefore, they falsely think the TSH test is the only test needed to diagnose thyroid disease.

When any test is discovered and marketed as the new gold standard, it tends to dull the critical thinking of doctors. When all the advertising and the doctors with the longest white coats say the test works, regular doctors begin to blindly accept the advertising as unquestionable truth and stop thinking for themselves. This sort of error has often happened in medicine—so often that you would think doctors would be wary of blindly trusting a patient's health to new tests. No research I know of has ever attempted to prove that the TSH test is the only test needed to check the state of your thyroid health, yet doctors keep acting as if it is the only thyroid test needed.

THE TAKE-HOME

Any time a test or treatment is called the *gold standard* in medicine, it tends to make doctors mentally lazy. This label leads them to think everything worth knowing about a topic is already known, and there is no need for further thought or effort. The TSH test is one such gold standard. The assumption that one test is sufficient for diagnosis and management often makes doctors look foolish, and causes patients to suffer. Doctors use the TSH test for everything from a physiological marker of thyroid function to a guide for initiating and monitoring thyroid medication dosages. It is an inadequate test for all these uses.

Most doctors have no idea how the normal range of a lab test is determined or what can falsely elevate or depress the measured level of a test. Before the TSH test became widely available, doctors listened to and examined their patients for symptoms and signs of thyroid disease. If a patient had severe fatigue, weight gain, and constipation and was losing the outer one-third of her eyebrows, doctors diagnosed the patient with hypothyroidism without needing the TSH test.

Now, because a gold standard has been announced for diagnosing thyroid issues, most doctors have stopped looking for physical signs and symptoms of thyroid disease. Instead, they only check a patient's TSH level instead. Another serious problem with this test is that the TSH level can be affected by a patient's smoking, sickness, stress level, or activity level (such as when the patient works out before having the lab work done). Most doctors have no idea that a patient's TSH level can be affected by so many things or that the level can change substantially over the course of a single day.

Whenever a patient makes time in a busy schedule to make an appointment with the doctor because fatigue, weight gain, mental cloudiness, and other symptoms have gotten so bad the patient can hardly function, doctors should listen to the symptoms and look for the signs of thyroid disease. In other words, the doctors should take the patients seriously. Next, the doctor should order a full thyroid panel that checks TSH, FT3, FT4, RT3, TPO, and TGA. There are several other non-thyroid tests the doctor needs to check to fully investigate possible thyroid problems. You can find the complete lists of tests in the book and website listed in the "Homework" section at the end of this chapter.

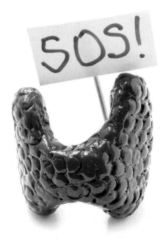

Many doctors have told patients that their thyroids were fine after a test returned a normal TSH value even though the patients have had serious thyroid disease and severe symptoms. When the TSH test is the only thyroid test the doctor checks, patients can have their TSH level come back *normal* for years before a doctor finally diagnoses them with thyroid disease. Many of these patients start taking an antidepressant pill. Some are told to exercise more and eat less, or they're told that their suffering is all in their head. I consider this very disrespectful and poor medical practice; it's malpractice, in fact.

To say the TSH test is the only test needed to diagnose thyroid disease is a lazy medical lie. If you have multiple thyroid symptoms, and a doctor has said that your *lab work* is normal, ask for a copy of the results to see what the doctor checked. (Your lab results belong to you, not to your doctor, so there's no reason you shouldn't be allowed to have a copy.) If the doctor and lab tested only the TSH, then you have the choice of going back to try to educate your doctor or finding a new doctor who will listen to you and take your symptoms seriously. Spend some time educating yourself using the two resources at the end of this chapter to learn about all the testing and thought doctors must do to provide an accurate diagnosis of thyroid disease.

DO AS I DO

Because thyroid symptoms can be rather subtle, I have my thyroid tested annually (if not more often). I don't stop with the TSH test; I check a full thyroid panel. I also make sure my wife has her levels checked. Thyroid health is closely linked with eating an organic, whole food diet and avoiding as many environmental toxins as possible, so that is how we eat and live.

HOMEWORK

It seems that most doctors refuse to do their homework on thyroid disease and thyroid testing, so you will have to do it for yourself. Here are two great places to begin learning about the complicated gland that is your thyroid.

BOOK: *The Paleo Thyroid Solution: Stop Feeling Fat, Foggy, and Fatigued at the Hands of Uninformed Doctors*
by Elle Russ (2016)

The author was a patient who was so mistreated by multiple doctors that she began a personal study and taught herself to treat her thyroid condition. This book includes an in-depth commentary from integrative physician Gary E. Foresman, MD.

WEBSITE: *StopTheThyroidMadness.com*
by Janie Bowthorpe

A couple of hours of reading and taking notes on this website will make you smarter than the average doctor is about hypothyroidism. The site also includes more than a decade's worth of patient experience with both testing and treatment of thyroid conditions.

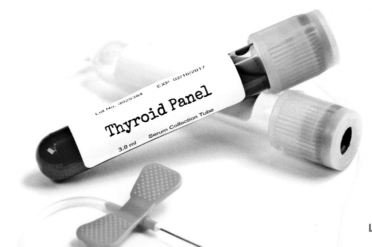

Chapter 17

IF YOU DON'T HAVE RICKETS, THEN YOUR VITAMIN D IS NORMAL

"

A smart mother makes often a better diagnosis than a poor doctor.

—August Bier

"

THE LIE

You get enough vitamin D from your diet. The fact that you don't have rickets (weak, bending bones in a child) or osteomalacia (weak, painful bones in an adult) is proof that you are getting enough vitamin D, and you don't need to take a vitamin D supplement.

WHY YOU SHOULD CARE

Vitamin D is not just a vitamin; it's a prohormone, which is an inactive hormone that must be activated in specific cells through a series of activation steps. It is involved in thousands of biochemical reactions in your body. If it does help your body in thousands of ways, and perhaps even prevents cancer, then you should make sure that you get enough vitamin D every day. If you need only enough vitamin D to prevent rickets and osteomalacia, then you are free to continue not caring about your vitamin D level.

There have been several small and medium research studies that demonstrate that getting more vitamin D could benefit health in many ways, but not many doctors seem to care. The USDA was content for decades to recommend the tiniest daily amount of vitamin D possible. Recently, the vitamin D RDA was increased by a small amount, and experts have started to recognize that different types of people (pregnant woman, children, and the elderly) need more vitamin D than other people. However, the current recommendation remains substandard for optimum health and disease prevention.

THE COMMON SENSE

Vitamin D is very important to hundreds of biochemical functions in the human body—so important, in fact, that our bodies learned thousands of years ago to make it from our exposure to sunlight. That seems like a pretty big deal. Over the last century, we have moved most of our activities indoors, out of the sun, and we've drastically cut the amount of fat we eat (fish oil, lard, and bacon are great sources of vitamin D), so our average vitamin D level has been steadily falling.

Vitamin D is responsible for so many beneficial things in the human body that it deserves a book of its own. Most of us know that vitamin D helps us absorb calcium to help keep our bones strong. However, an increasing number of experts are starting to recognize that this may be the least of its benefits. Vitamin D appears to have great benefits for your immune system, mood, heart health, and even sexual function. It is becoming clear that taking the minimal amount to keep rickets and osteomalacia away isn't sufficient for optimal health.

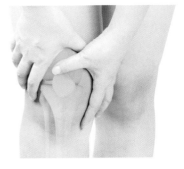

THE RESEARCH

There are two groups of thought, and two types of research on this topic. One set of experts focuses only on the minimal amount of vitamin D needed to avoid severe deficiency. These experts focused their research on this topic, and they didn't do research studies that involved taking more than 1,000 daily IU. (IU stands for international units, which is the measurement unit for vitamin D.) These studies are what medical schools teach; therefore most practicing doctors know only about these minimum requirements.

More recently, another set of researchers have found that higher levels of vitamin D can be very beneficial for many different areas of human health. Research studies and reviews have shown a correlation between higher vitamin D intake and reduced rates of cancer, type 1 diabetes, multiple sclerosis, skin cancer, and other diseases. The literature suggests that it's very hard to harm yourself by taking too much vitamin D. One case study followed an individual who accidentally took more than 100,000 IU daily (from a mislabeled supplement) for months. Although he suffered nausea and body aches while taking this much vitamin D, as soon as he discovered his overdose and discontinued taking that quantity, he went right back to normal with no long-term consequences.

THE TAKE-HOME

In 2007, I read an article about vitamin D that stated there was a rampant vitamin D deficiency in most people. I didn't find this article in a respected medical journal. I found it on an alternative health website. I was very skeptical of this information because I hadn't read anything about this deficiency in more official medical literature. To do some research on my own, I started checking vitamin D-25 levels (not the 1,25 level) in some of my older patients, who were at risk of osteoporosis. Vitamin D-25 is a much more accurate test and is the only one that should be checked.

To my surprise, I found that seventy-two patients out of one hundred had a vitamin D-25 level below 30 ng/mL. Normal is 30 ng/mL to 100 ng/mL. In my opinion, the optimal level is 50 ng/mL to 100 ng/mL. That means that a total of 72 percent of my elderly patients were deficient in this vital substance, and I had been completely unaware of the situation! I hadn't been taught about the importance of checking vitamin D-25 levels and was blind to the deficiency in my patients. I began ordering vitamin D-25 levels for younger and younger patients, and I found many of them also were deficient in vitamin D. I was mortified by this discovery, and I immediately read everything I could find about vitamin D. I began recommending that all my patients take a vitamin D3 (not vitamin D2) supplement.

I spoke to several of my doctor friends about my discovery. They told me that they never checked vitamin D levels in their patients, and they seemingly had no interest in starting to test. The more I read about vitamin D, the more I was convinced that it was a vital ingredient for overall health. However, I felt like a lone voice in the wilderness. Most patients would have no idea why they should take vitamin D because the media had never covered this issue, and other doctors wouldn't have brought it up. In some cases, I had patients whom I had referred to various specialists come back to see me who reported that the specialist had told them to stop taking the vitamin

D supplement I had recommended. The specialists said the patients didn't need the supplements and might experience a dangerous overdose.

These specialists usually offered this *advice* without checking the patients' vitamin D levels. The doctors didn't base the recommendations on research or critical thinking. When I did more investigation into the research on vitamin D overdoses, I discovered that not one serious overdose had ever been reported. None. Zero. Zip. Zilch. Although people had accidentally significantly exceeded the RDA for long periods of time, there was not a single death or serious injury. So, if your doctor warns you against taking more than 1,000 IU of vitamin D, you can be sure he has read nothing new on the subject since he was in medical school.

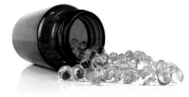

DO AS I DO

As I said in an earlier chapter, I play in the sun without sunscreen as often as possible. I eat lots of pastured fatty foods like butter, egg yolks, and pork. I also take 5,000 to 10,000 IU of vitamin D3 every day as needed to keep my level above 50. I check the vitamin D level in my blood twice yearly, and the results show I am not close to overdosing. I will always take a daily vitamin D supplement unless I move closer to the equator where the sun is stronger.

HOMEWORK

There are several books about vitamin D therapy, how much you should take, and why supplementing vitamin D is important. However, I'm recommending a website because it's a great place to start your vitamin D education. Armed with this information from this site, you can discuss your vitamin D needs with your doctor.

WEBSITE: *Vitamin D Resource Page* The Vitamin D Council
Visit http://bit.ly/VitDFAQ for a very useful resource for learning about vitamin D and all of its powers to prevent and heal.

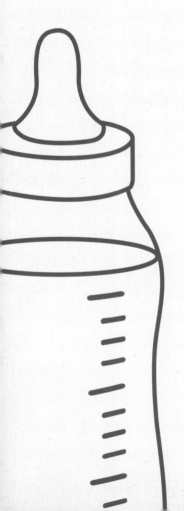

Chapter 18

BREAST MILK

DOESN'T CONTAIN EVERYTHING A NEWBORN NEEDS?

66

It is important to keep in mind that our bodies must work pretty well, or there wouldn't be so many humans on the planet.

—Ina May Gaskin

THE LIE

Human breast milk is deficient in vitamin D. Babies who are exclusively breastfed should be given vitamin D drops.

WHY YOU SHOULD CARE

We want our babies to receive the best nutrition possible to give them a head start on a healthy, happy life. If breast milk is truly deficient in vitamin D, then we should give vitamin D drops to babies who are exclusively breastfed. If breast milk contains everything a baby needs, then let's not tell new mothers that their breast milk is deficient and that Big Pharma needs to help nourish the babies.

SUPPORT FOR THE LIE

Every medical and nursing student has been taught this medical lie for as long as any of us can remember. Studies that examine the nutrition in breast milk did indeed show it had almost no vitamin D at all. With this seemingly straightforward information, it seemed clear that infants who were to be exclusively breastfed should receive supplemental vitamin D drops to make up for this shortfall. This lie is ingrained in medical education and will probably take decades to erase.

THE COMMON SENSE

One of my first *what-the-hell?* moments in medical school came when I heard this lie. I've always been of the opinion that the Creator and Mother Nature have taken care of everything. The job of doctors is to correct the little errors that occasionally happen and fix the trauma we humans inflict upon ourselves. My memory is that my medical team (which was our attending physician, a senior resident, two interns, and three of us lowly medical students) was on the labor and delivery ward one early morning. We had been on call all night, delivering babies and assisting with cesarean sections. All of us were exhausted. The intern was presenting a patient's information to the team and was going over the baby's regimen.

He mentioned vitamin D drops. One of the medical students (not me—I was too tired to ask questions that day) asked why the newborn was getting these drops. The senior resident, who was annoyed by all medical students, told us that all babies needed vitamin D drops because there is no vitamin D in breast milk. This statement woke me up. I glanced at our attending physician, who I was sure would correct the resident, but he only nodded in quiet agreement. "How can that be?" I thought to myself, although I was too tired to speak out. When did mothers stop putting vitamin D in their breast milk? I was about to ask that question, but by that time we had moved on to the next patient. I filed the question away for later research. Although I didn't have time to research the issue then, I kept returning to the thought. Something about it just didn't seem right.

Vitamin D drops have been around for less than one hundred years, so it makes one wonder how humans could have survived for thousands of years without giving breastfed babies (which would have been all babies for centuries) vitamin D drops. Maybe vitamin D is not that important? No, research continues to show that it's vital to thousands of biochemical reactions in the bodies of babies and adults. It is both a prohormone and a vitamin. We must have this essential substance, so how did babies obtain vitamin D in the days before the invention of vitamin D drops? Were mothers of the past somehow able to produce vitamin D in their breast milk, whereas modern moms had lost this ability? It turns out that *is* the explanation, and the reason seems obvious when you know it.

THE RESEARCH

As I said earlier, about seventy years ago, research started showing that human breast milk contained almost no vitamin D. This discovery has never been disputed, and apparently decades passed before anyone questioned the reason. However, Professor Bruce Hollis, PhD, thought he might have a theory about why mothers seemingly let their infants down in such an important way. He decided to give breastfeeding mothers supplemental vitamin D to see if the supplements would enable them to produce vitamin D in their milk. Hollis began by giving the mothers 2,400 IU of vitamin D daily (much more than the RDA for breastfeeding mothers). Even after supplementing with this seemingly high amount, the

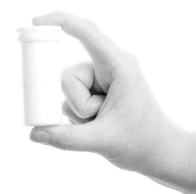

mothers still produced so little vitamin D in their milk that the ethics committee stopped the study for the safety of the infants.

Hollis then decided to give the mothers 6,400 IU of vitamin D daily, and, amazingly, the mothers in the study started excreting vitamin D in their milk! In fact, they produced so much vitamin D in their milk that their infants didn't need the supplemental drops. They were getting everything they needed from their mothers, just as it should be. Hollis published his study in 2015, and it should have jerked the entire medical community awake, but it did not. Very few obstetricians, pediatricians, or family doctors even know about this study, much less use its results to counsel their patients. This study was large, well-managed, randomized, and double-blinded. There can be no doubt about the truth of its findings, yet the results are helping very few patients.

THE TAKE-HOME

Breast milk is more than a liquid; it is a living tissue custom formulated by each mother for her baby. Hundreds of years ago, breastfeeding mothers got plenty of vitamin D from the sun and their high-fat diets. Therefore, they produced plenty of vitamin D in their breast milk for their babies. My feeling about this had been right all along. When the female body has proper nourishment and exposure to the sun, it will produce every single vitamin, mineral, and nutrient an infant needs to grow and succeed. The reason why the previously mentioned studies had shown low levels of vitamin D in human breast milk was because those modern women, who lived indoors and ate lower-fat foods, had very low levels of vitamin D in their blood. They were, therefore, not able to produce more for the breast milk for their babies.

I'm still flabbergasted when I think of the intelligent professors and doctors who taught my classes at the university. Why had none of them ever thought about, or questioned, this seeming deficiency in the makeup of breast milk? They were evidently too busy and/or not willing to make negative waves by questioning the traditional teaching. Every day, doctors are busy interacting with an endless cycle of miraculous biochemical events in human metabolism. Doctors are used to the human body healing itself, growing, reproducing, and doing many other amazing things. Why would doctors be comfortable thinking that this same human body might forget how to produce one of the most important vitamins in human breast milk?

This lack of logic should have immediately raised red flags about the deficient amount of vitamin D in the mothers' diets, but it didn't. As usual, instead of fixing the underlying problem or deficiency, doctors and Big Pharma decided to prescribe vitamin D drops to the infant to fix the problem. But what if a mother couldn't afford the drops or didn't want to administer them for the time she was exclusively breastfeeding her baby? Wouldn't it have been more elegant to give the mother the right amount of vitamin D? Then, not only would the mother have had the vitamin D she needed for her body but she could have effortlessly passed vitamin D to her baby every time she breastfed. Instead, we find ourselves in a situation in which busy mothers often forget to get the drops at the pharmacy or forget to give the drops to their babies every day. Thus, their babies have an increased risk of diseases, such as rickets. When these babies are grown up, they will most certainly suffer from vitamin D deficiency.

Any time experts say that human bodies don't make or do something we need, we should be immediately suspicious. Unless they can convincingly explain why this is the case, you should start doing research for yourself. Women who are trying to get pregnant should take 6,000 to 8,000 IU of vitamin D daily from the time they start trying to conceive until the day after they wean their baby from breast milk. That supplementation will take care of the baby's needs. Since the modern diet is currently so deficient in vitamin D, all of us should probably take that amount every day regardless of whether we're breastfeeding a child.

DO AS I DO

I get excited every time I explain to one of my pregnant patients that if she takes a vitamin D supplement, then she can make everything her new baby needs to thrive and be healthy. Make sure any of your friends or family who are with child know they can make everything their baby needs. A baby doesn't need anything a mother can't provide.

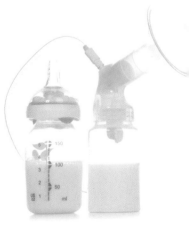

HOMEWORK

Once you understand this topic, it's such a no-brainer that no further study is needed. I think you deserve the day off from homework.

Chapter 19

GOD MADE THE SUN, AND GOD MADE YOU

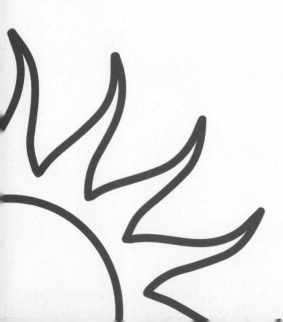

"

I think you might dispense
with half your doctors if
you would only consult
Dr. Sun more.

—Henry Ward Beecher

"

THE LIE

Exposure to sunlight causes skin cancer. To decrease the risk of skin cancer, you should stay out of the sun as much as possible. If you must be in the sun, then you should wear lots of high-SPF sunscreen to protect yourself. You should even wear sunscreen when you're inside if you will be exposed to sunlight from windows.

WHY YOU SHOULD CARE

Any time medical science tells you to avoid nature or something natural, your BS sensor should sound an alarm. If we're now considering the sun to be dangerous, you should protect yourself from it, and there better be some darn good research to back up this claim. However, if there is no meaningful research to support this "dangerous sun theory," then you may continue to play in the sun and use it to make vitamin D as humans have done for thousands of years.

SUPPORT FOR THE LIE

The American Society for Dermatologic Surgery (ASDS) and the American Academy of Dermatology (AAD), the two leading academies of skin doctors in the United States, have an endless supply of brochures that repeat this medical lie. These societies recommend that you wear sunscreen to prevent skin cancer (even indoors!). You can find thousands of pages of "patient education" on this topic on the societies' websites.

Almost every doctor you ask tells you to limit your sun exposure and to wear sunscreen whenever you will be in the sun; in some cases, doctors say to avoid sunlight altogether. Some studies seem to show a link between sun exposure and certain types of skin cancer. However, most of these studies are poorly designed (for example, one was done on donated baby foreskins that were no longer attached to the baby), or the conclusion of the study does not logically follow from its findings.

THE COMMON SENSE

Humans have been playing and working in the sunshine for many thousands of years. Sunlight is as natural as, well... sunlight! Making the claim that exposure to sunlight causes cancer would require exactly the same stretch of the imagination as saying that drinking pure mountain spring water causes cancer or that eating organic green plants causes cancer. Human skin has been exposed to sunlight for so long that it has learned to use sunlight to make a vitamin/prohormone (vitamin D).

Despite these facts, a few decades ago doctors *discovered* that somehow the sun is dangerous to human skin, and we should protect our skin from the sun's damaging effects. On the commonsense level, this lie is ridiculous. In our modern society, in which we often believe things that make no sense and repeat them as truth, this lie has caught traction and become the official stance of the skin specialists. It has become the mantra of skin-care experts everywhere. From dermatologists to sunscreen makers, everyone who can make a living promoting the dangerous sun theory is doing so.

For thousands of years, no one gave a second thought to sunshine being the cause of any disease. However, in the last forty years, some of the smartest among us have *discovered* that the very thing that makes all life on Earth possible is now also the leading cause of skin cancer. Life wouldn't exist on Earth if it were not for the sun, so it strains believability that this same sun is now dangerous to life.

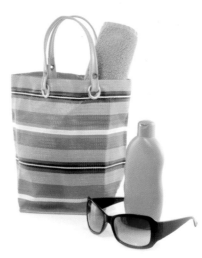

THE RESEARCH

There is no major scientific study that proves conclusively that exposure to sunlight causes skin cancer. You're probably thinking, *"What?!* There must be some research that proves this lie true. Otherwise, doctors wouldn't keep repeating it, right?"

There are several kinds of skin cancer. The most dangerous and worrisome by far is melanoma. If sunlight exposure increases the risk of melanoma, it would be easy to prove with scientific studies showing that you are more likely to get skin cancer on your face or other areas of your skin that receive the most sun exposure. However, this has not been the case. Melanoma is often on areas of the skin that experience minimal sun exposure or no sun exposure at all. There is no research proving that melanoma is more likely to occur at sites of repeated sun exposure. This one fact alone should cause doctors to rethink their sun-blocking advice.

As we've started to use more sunscreen and wear more hats and long-sleeved shirts to block the sun, researchers should have been able to detect a decline in the rates of melanoma. However, the research shows that rates of melanoma have increased in the past decade.

Every research study cited by the AAD or the ASDS contains flaws in the method, number of participants in the study, or the conclusions drawn from the results. If another researcher attempted to use the same study design to prove that sunlight does *not* cause cancer, the AAD and the ASDS would have a field day discrediting that study because of its fatally flawed study design. Your doctor's job is to dig into research and prove to himself that the conclusions are valid before he gives you advice based on a study. Unfortunately, doctors seldom spend the time to make an effort to do this.

The sad truth of how things usually work in the real world is that a primary care doctor sees a news story on television reporting that the National Academy of Super Geniuses has decided that Something causes Another Thing, and Everyone should avoid that Something. With no research or real thought, this doctor then starts recommending to his patients that they avoid Something. This doctor might also skim the first couple of paragraphs of an article in a medical journal about this Something-causes-Another Thing topic. Based on his cursory inspection of the article, he still concludes that he should tell his patients to avoid that Something. Unfortunately, that doctor doesn't bother to read how the researchers conducted the study, the number of participants in the study, or if the conclusion matches the findings, which is all information he needs to make a good assessment about what his recommendation should be.

You might be surprised to learn that there's a sizable amount of research demonstrating that sunshine actually reduces certain kinds of skin cancer, as well as cancer in other parts of the body. One large study showed that people who work outside in the sun are less likely to get skin cancer than indoor workers. (Yes, you read that right.) Another large study shows that living further from the equator is a risk factor for skin cancer and other types of cancers. (Yes, you also read that correctly.) Because these studies don't support the popular expert opinion of the moment, they get little traction with doctors or the news media; therefore, you might have never heard of them.

Here's the important question we should all be asking: Why are we only researching putting chemicals on the skin and/or avoiding the sun to decrease skin cancer? For instance, why are we not researching whether it matters what our skin is made of? In other words, someone should research whether the things we eat and drink increase our risk of skin cancer. Could it be that eating quality natural foods would help you build better skin that is much less likely to become cancerous? If you look at a map that shows the geographical variation in melanoma incidence, you might be struck by two things, first, melanoma occurs much more frequently in locations with weaker sunlight, and secondly, it occurs much more frequently in areas of the world that tend to eat a standard Western diet of highly processed sugars, grains, and vegetable/seed oils.

Geographical Variation in Melanoma Incidence

Cutaneous melanoma incidence
(per 100,000 individuals)

- 4.1+
- 1.8–4.1
- 0.89–1.8
- 0.48–0.89
- <0.48
- No data

Equator

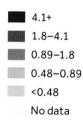

I've had many patients tell me an interesting thing: They found that after they had decreased the amount of grains and vegetable oils in their diets and had started eating more colorful berries and veggies, they could spend more time in the sun without burning. A few patients who experienced severe reactions to the sun in the past were happily surprised to find that they no longer had these reactions after they started eating an improved whole food diet. So, why are medical scientists not interested in investigating whether there are things in our diet that increase rates of skin cancer?

The sun hasn't changed at all in the past fifty years, as we will discuss shortly. The ozone layer has changed a little in the last fifty years, but the average human diet has changed almost completely in the past 50 years. That sounds like an important place for researchers to look, if you ask me.

THE TAKE-HOME

So what should we make of all this? How can we think about this problem in a way that honors our extensive experience as a species on this planet while balancing it with what doctors are currently telling us? We have been told that the increase in skin cancer over the past few decades is because the ozone layer is getting thinner, which means it lets in more ultraviolet (UV) light. However, there is a major problem with that theory.

If you start at the North Pole, where the sun's rays are very weak, and travel south toward to the equator, the UV exposure you would receive from the sun along the way would increase by more than 5,000 percent as you near the equator. People who live along the equator in places like Ecuador, Brazil, and Kenya, regardless of skin tone, receive many thousands of times the UV radiation as people who live in the far north in places such as Norway, Canada, and Russia. For the increased UV radiation that enters our atmosphere through a thinning ozone layer to be the cause of the skin cancer epidemic, wouldn't the UV levels need to be increased by an amount greater than the naturally occurring increase one would encounter while traveling from the far north toward the equator? Ozone depletion during the past fifty years has been reported by leading climate scientists to have increased UV exposure by, at most, 20 percent. This is a minuscule percentage compared to the large increase in UV exposure caused merely by traveling from Canada to Brazil. This fact alone should cause every doctor to reevaluate what he believes about this topic. The UV exposure from the sun because of ozone depletion has barely changed, yet we have a growing skin cancer epidemic. What else could possibly be to blame?

Your skin is made of what you eat. Your skin is completely replaced with new skin cells every month or two, and the new cells are made of the proteins, fats, and other nutrients you have eaten, for better or for worse. Therefore, what has changed over the past fifty years that could lead to these increasing rates of skin cancer? We've established that the sun hasn't really changed. And the ozone layer has changed a tiny amount, but not nearly enough to account for our skin cancer epidemic. How much have our food choices and food quality changed over the past fifty years? A heck of a lot.

During this past century, our species has gone from eating a mostly organic, vegetable-rich food supply grown by local farmers to eating a mass-produced, grain-heavy food supply that is grown, harvested, and processed by large corporations. Our diet is much higher in sugar, grains, and vegetable oils, not to mention questionable chemicals that are added, either accidentally or on purpose, during manufacturing. Why does no doctor ever stop to consider this as it relates to skin cancer?

The building blocks that our body receives for building our skin (and performing other functions) have changed. In the meantime, all doctors focus on telling patients to avoid the sun, to slather our skin with expensive protective products, and to have an expensive medical procedure to remove a piece of damaged skin. On the AAD's skin cancer prevention web page, there is no reference to how your diet might be related to your risk of skin cancer. This is a shame. Why is a website seemingly dedicated to skin health passing up on such a wonderful opportunity to educate people on how important a proper diet is in the prevention of skin cancer?

Are we doctors really so simpleminded that we need to think, "Because the sun shines on the skin, then skin cancer must be the sun's fault"? If you built the roof of your house with shoddy materials, and it collapsed after a few years, did sun exposure on the roof cause the collapse, or were the building supplies you used to build the roof to blame? Part of the explanation for this seeming simplemindedness is how companies make money for *preventing* skin cancer, and how doctors are paid for treating skin cancer.

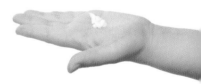

Companies are paid to develop products that block the sun. There are now hundreds of different kinds of sunscreens on the market. The more blockage they provide (the higher the SPF), the more they cost. If a company develops a sunscreen that is better, easier to use, cheaper to purchase, and so on, then the company's profits increase. A company would make very little profit at all by telling people to stop eating junk food. The same concept applies to how doctors are paid to treat and remove skin cancers.

Insurance pays a doctor about the same amount for a routine office visit as they pay to remove a noncancerous skin lesion. For removing a precancerous skin lesion (*actinic keratosis*), the doctor is paid roughly twice the amount that's paid for an office visit. Therefore, just by *calling* a skin lesion a precancerous lesion, a doctor can double what he is paid to remove it. If the lesion is diagnosed as cancer, with or without a pathologist confirming the diagnosis, the doctor is paid anywhere from four times the cost of an office visit fee up to many times more to remove that lesion.

If the doctor removes a large enough piece of skin, the patient also needs expensive skin grafting procedures to repair the defect, and, of course, that's another charge. You can easily see how it's in the doctor's financial best interest for your skin lesion to be labeled precancerous or skin cancer. The same doctor who makes the precancerous or skin cancer diagnosis would have been paid very little to counsel you years earlier to avoid eating grains or using vegetable oils in cooking and to include certain vitamins in your diet to prevent skin cancer from ever starting in the first place.

Before you gallantly jump to your doctor's defense and say that he would never stoop so low as to misdiagnose a skin lesion, consider this. The diagnosing of a skin lesion as something worse than it actually is has become so common that the practice has a name; an article in the *British Journal of Dermatology* calls this practice *diagnostic drift*. This article reveals diagnostic drift to be a significant cause of the skin cancer epidemic that we have been hearing about over the past few decades. If a doctor's prestige and income depend upon a skin lesion being cancer, then, more often than not, that lesion will be diagnosed as cancer. Refer to Chapter 2 to understand why this is not necessarily caused by dishonesty or some kind of conspiracy. It is just human nature.

I know this chapter has given you a lot to think about and question. I'm also aware that dermatologists will not be thrilled with me for having spilled these particular beans. However, my duty is to my patients and to you, dear reader. If I, as other doctors have done, ignore common sense and blame something as natural as the sun for this skin cancer epidemic, then I am a part of the problem. My plan, however, is to be part of the solution, come what may.

DO AS I DO

I eat many servings of colorful veggies every day, take my vitamins, and play in the sun all I want. I rarely use sunscreen. I have a fair complexion, so I still burn if I stay in the sun too long, and I try never to do that. Sunburns that cause peeling hurt, and that kind of extreme sun exposure might be what leads to an increased skin cancer risk.

When I ate a processed, grain-based, junk-food diet, I sunburned easily and terribly after only a short time in the sun. I probably had a much higher risk of skin cancer back then as well. Talk to your doctor about the real causes of skin cancer, and make sure to read and research. You can then decide how you and your family will work and play in the sun to keep your skin healthy.

HOMEWORK

The homework for this chapter is more involved than what I've assigned in other chapters. I want you to email the AAD (www.aad.org/Forms/ContactUs/Default.aspx) and the ASDS (www.asds.net/Skin-Experts/Contact-ASDS) and ask to have copies of the research studies that prove that sun exposure leads to skin cancer. Ignore the BS, bluff, and bluster you will receive in reply and look only at the facts. You are likely to get a stack of brochures stating the societies' official opinions and positions, but you probably won't receive any actual research studies. Then, the next time you're at your doctor's office, ask him the same question. Tell him to take his time and find the most powerful study he can that shows the link between sun exposure and skin cancer and email a copy to you.

You will be amazed, and perhaps disappointed, at the dodging and subject-changing that takes place. Don't be tricked or dissuaded; be respectfully persistent. If you receive an email containing a study, read it carefully and research it. I think you will discover the actual findings in any study sent to you will be lacking and lame and not worthy of making you fear something as natural as sunlight.

Chapter 20

FIBER IS NECESSARY FOR A HEALTHY GUT

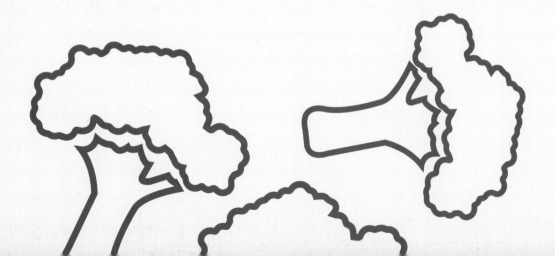

No organ in the body is so misunderstood, so slandered and maltreated as the colon.

—Sir Arthur Hurst

THE LIE

Fiber is good for you, and you should try to get as much fiber in your diet as possible. Fiber will help with constipation and irritable bowel syndrome (IBS). Fiber will help prevent diverticulitis and probably even colon cancer.

WHY YOU SHOULD CARE

If fiber is vital for gut health then you should eat lots of it. However, if fiber is actually irritating to your gut, as several studies show, then you should probably limit your fiber intake, especially if you have IBS or diverticulosis.

SUPPORT FOR THE LIE

Everyone, from your parents to your doctor to your dietitian, is quick to tell you that fiber is good for you. The Big Food industry also loves repeating this lie because it's easy for them to add a little fiber to whatever junk they're trying to sell you, and they then put a "high-fiber" label on the box. People will tell you that getting extra fiber will prevent constipation, diverticulosis, and even colon cancer. There are several observational studies based on self-reported Food Frequency Questionnaire (FFQ) data that seem to support this hypothesis. The problem is, there are no randomized controlled trials (RCT) that show any of this to be true.

Although the observational studies seem to show a correlation between increased fiber intake and decreased rates of constipation, diverticulosis, and colon cancer, an observational study does not prove causation. The observational studies counted the dietary fiber from vegetables and fruit rather than from the fiber the food industry adds to junk food.

THE COMMON SENSE

Fiber is undigestible plant matter that passes through the digestive tract and is expelled unchanged in the feces. You can often see high-fiber foods in the toilet, unchanged in appearance from when you ate them. The Institute of Medicine currently recommends a daily fiber intake of 38 grams for men and 25 grams for women.

If you see a group of firefighters in the front yard of a house, it is highly likely that the house is burning. This does not mean the firefighters caused the fire; they are merely associated with the fire. The firefighters' presence in the yard proves correlation but not causation. In the same respect, the fact that eating more fibrous vegetables and fruits is correlated with decreased risks of colon/bowel problems does not prove that the fiber is preventing those conditions.

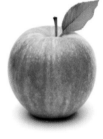

Most people who include many fiber-filled vegetables and fruit in their diet also eat diets that are healthier overall, and they live healthier lives. They are less likely to smoke, drink alcohol heavily, or eat lots of processed junk food. In many of the studies, these confounding variables are not controlled for, and thus may be the cause of the increased risk of colon/bowel disease rather than the lack of fiber.

For most of their existence on this planet, humans ate lots of fatty meat and a few vegetables. They certainly ate berries, fruits, and honey when they could get them, but this was rare. There is no evidence that our ancestors went out of their way to eat extra fiber.

THE RESEARCH

Virtually all the research suggesting that eating more fiber is good for you is in the form of prospective, observational studies, which don't prove causation. This is not sufficient evidence for a doctor or dietitian to tell patients to eat more fiber. When controlled studies are done on the topics of constipation, diverticulosis, and colon cancer, adding more fiber to the diet has no effect whatsoever on the outcome of the study.

One review article, which looked at multiple studies that investigated whether fiber played a role in the treatment of chronic constipation, found that the less fiber the participants ate, the fewer symptoms of constipation they had. You read that correctly. The participants who ate the most fiber had more severe constipation symptoms than those in the study who ate no fiber at all.

Two large studies seemed to show no colon health benefits from eating more dietary fiber. The Nurses Health Study followed 88,757 women for years and found no increased risk of colon cancer in the women who ate the least fiber. The Health Professionals Follow-Up Study followed 47,949 men for years and also found no difference in colon cancer rates between the men who ate the most fiber versus those who ate the least fiber.

THE TAKE-HOME

As with all dietary topics, we should look to our past to understand what we should eat in the present. Although it is known that our ancestors would travel great distances to acquire certain nutrients (such as salt), there is no evidence that our ancestors went out of their way to get extra fiber. Fiber is an indigestible irritant to our bowels, and it can act as an antinutrient, preventing absorption of some vitamins and minerals we need. If I told you to eat a cup of sawdust (full of fiber) each day in order to keep your bowels healthy, cancer-free, and moving regularly, you might think I was crazy. But, the fiber many experts recommend that we eat actually contains sawdust (or wood fibers that are very much like sawdust). This recommendation does not square with how our ancestors ate. Until some good, controlled research proves the advice to eat more fiber to be correct, experts should stop advising their patients to do so.

There are people, and other animals, who eat a Carnivore diet (all meat—no plant matter at all—and zero grams of fiber) for years at a time. These people report no constipation and no increased risk of diverticulosis or colon cancer.

Any fiber you eat should come from whole, unprocessed vegetables and never from factory-added fiber that's in junk food. Any possible good you would get from eating added fiber (from sawdust or grains) is offset by the inflammatory properties those additives would produce. The worst possible source of fiber is a bowl of highly processed grain cereal with added pseudofiber.

DO AS I DO

I never go out of my way to eat extra fiber. In fact, there are many days each week when I eat no fiber at all. I believe humans have eaten mostly fatty meat for thousands of years, and I try to mimic

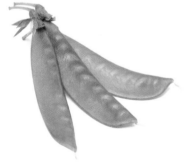

this way of eating. I occasionally eat some vegetables, but what I eat seldom contains more than a few grams of fiber.

Even though I eat very little fiber, if any, each day, I have no problems in the restroom, no pain, no cramping. It might be that some people need some small amount of fiber in their diet to prevent constipation issues, but I am not one of them.

HOMEWORK

This lie has reached such mythological proportions that it will likely take years for the average person to begin to understand the truth about added fiber. Big Food makes billions of dollars from highly processed added-fiber foods, so the manufacturers will certainly be pumping the brakes of paradigm shift as often as they can. Here are a couple of resources to help you start to make sense of this topic.

BLOG POST: *"A Carnivorous Diet"* by Amber O'Hearn on the Empirica website (2012) at http://bit.ly/NoFiber

Long-time carnivore Amber O'Hearn breaks down the science and practical results of a fiber-free diet.

PAPER: *"Myths and Misconceptions About Chronic Constipation"* by Stefan A. Müller-Lissner (2005) at http://bit.ly/ChronicConstipation

The article discusses classic myths (lies) about what does and does not cause constipation.

BLOG POST: *World Carnivore Tribe* at http://bit.ly/ CarnivoreTribe

This Facebook group has more than 25,000 members at this time. Here you can read the stories of thousands of happy people who have been fiber-free for years, and you can ask them your questions.

Chapter 21
EATING RED MEAT CAUSES CANCER

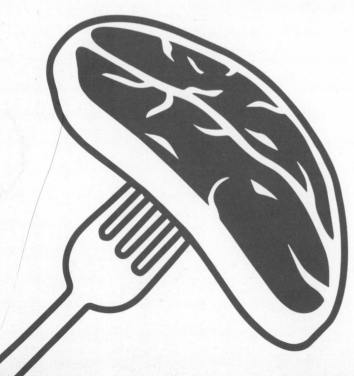

66

The soul becomes dyed with the color of its thoughts.

—Marcus Aurelius

99

THE LIE

Red meat is not good for you, and eating more than a single small serving daily will increase your risk of colon cancer or increase your cancer risk overall.

WHY YOU SHOULD CARE

If eating red meat increases your risk of developing cancer, then you should avoid it. However, if red meat does not cause cancer, you should eat lots of red meat to take advantage of all the nutrition it contains. There is no question that red meat is filled with vitamins, minerals, protein, and healthy fats.

SUPPORT FOR THE LIE

The World Health Organization (WHO) has proclaimed red meat to be a probable cause of cancer in humans. Due to this risk, the WHO advises that humans limit red meat in their diets. The recommendation is based on a few prospective observational studies that showed a slight correlation between eating red meat and increased risk of cancer. The data for these studies came from self-reported data collected on Food Frequency Questionnaires (FFQs).

All the experts on this subject bluster and blow about the absolute truth of this lie, but the actual research is quite anemic. Not a single controlled study proves any link between eating red meat and increased cancer risk.

THE COMMON SENSE

Humans, in our present form, have been eating red meat for at least 200,000 years. Long before we cultivated grain, fermented wine, or made cheese, we were hunting large animals and eating their meat. Our ancestors hunted many species of large animals to extinction. To now say that the red meat that has nourished us for millennia has become bad for us seems silly from a commonsense standpoint.

Our species flourished and prospered by eating the meat of large mammals. Indeed, some experts believe the reason our brain size increased to its current size is because of the quantities of fatty red meat our ancestors consumed. So, if science is going to tell us that a food that has nourished us for so long is now bad for us, there'd better be some hard data to back up that claim.

THE RESEARCH

As with other lies I've discussed, the research to support the lie that red meat is a probable cause of cancer comes from poorly conducted epidemiological studies, which show correlation between two things rather than proving that one thing causes the other. Most of these observational studies are based on those food frequency questionnaires that contain self-reported data from the research participants. Questions such as, "How many cups of ribs have you consumed in the past 3 months?" are difficult to answer, and participants are likely to guess or estimate to come up with a response.

Another problem with this kind of research is the researcher's preconceived ideas. Because this type of study is neither randomized nor double-blinded, the preconceived notions of the researcher can seep into the results of the study, and very often do. This bias is not evidence of dishonesty; it's just human nature to see what you are expecting to find.

Fear of judgment can keep study participants from telling the complete truth. If the respondents think someone is going to be reading the results making judgments about the answers, they might very well fudge on their answers one way or another. Researchers are unable to control for this reaction from participants, so the FFQs typically yield little useful information.

Confounders are other things that could be leading to the outcome the study is looking for. For example, many people who eat lots of red meat also smoke and drink alcohol, both of which increase cancer risk. If these types of variables are not controlled for in the study, they can skew the results and give false conclusions. Many studies that seem to show a link between red meat and cancer did not control for smoking, alcohol intake, or activity level. Not adjusting the data for such confounders renders the results of the study useless.

It's true that the link between smoking and lung cancer was deduced from epidemiological studies, but smokers showed a 15 to 30 times greater risk of lung cancer than nonsmokers. Although the results didn't prove that smoking causes cancer, the high relative risk makes it very likely to be a cause. In the case of the epidemiological research linking red meat to cancer risk, the results showed barely 1.5 times greater risk. Most researchers don't even pay attention to relative risks lower than 2, and the red meat–to-cancer link just doesn't make the cut.

THE TAKE-HOME

Given the very long history of humanity eating all the red meat it could hunt down and kill (we drove several large species to extinction), it seems unlikely that eating red meat leads to anything other than good health. If red meat truly causes cancer, then it seems possible that humans should already be extinct because of all the cancer our ancestors would have had from eating all that red meat. There is no evidence in anthropology or archeology that our ancestors considered red meat to be anything other than a delicious, healthy food.

When we stop depending on newspaper headlines for our scientific knowledge on this topic and actually dig down into the research, we come away with very little evidence that red meat causes cancer. Researchers who truly believe this should design some better studies that will show a convincing link between red meat and cancer.

DO AS I DO

Red meat is a large part of my daily keto-carnivore diet. I eat red meat grilled, smoked, fried, and roasted. I have no fear that red meat will make me anything other than very healthy, just like it did for my ancestors. Red meat cooked over an open flame nourished my ancestors for thousands of centuries, and it nourishes me as well. I keep an eye on the research, but so far I've seen nothing that makes me fear enjoying the nutrition in red meat.

HOMEWORK

There are groups who would prefer you eat a plant-based diet and not eat animal-sourced foods. They include the vegan-vegetarian groups, Big Food, and Big Pharma. The vegan/vegetarian groups believe it is morally wrong for humans to eat other animals, even though we've done so for millennia. Big Food makes millions of dollars through manufacturing processed plant-based food products, so their motivation is clear. Big Pharma, as is often usual, is currently so confused and misguided about this topic that its motivation is unclear.

BOOK: *Eat Meat and Stop Jogging: "Common" Advice on How to Get Fit Is Keeping You Fat and Making You Sick* by Mike Sheridan (2014)

This book is about the benefits of eating a meat-heavy diet. And it suggests you stop jogging if you hate it, like I do.

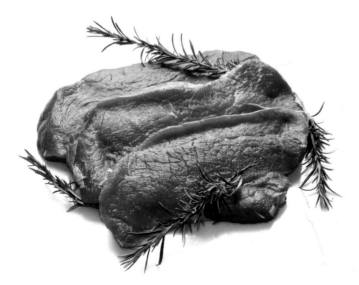

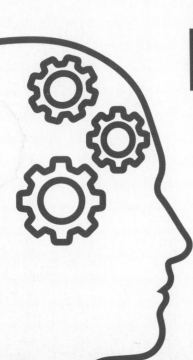

Chapter 22

YOU MUST EAT LOTS OF CARBOHYDRATES TO FUEL YOUR BRAIN

"

Whenever a doctor cannot do good, he must be kept from doing harm.

—Hippocrates

"

THE LIE

You must eat plenty of carbohydrates each day, or your brain and other body parts will not have enough energy to function properly.

WHY YOU SHOULD CARE

If eating carbohydrates is essential to proper brain and body function, then you should eat lots of carbohydrates at each meal. However, if you don't need carbohydrates to power the brain and other organs, and they lead to increased levels of blood glucose and insulin, then you should limit them.

SUPPORT FOR THE LIE

It seems most doctors and dietitians will repeat this lie effortlessly. It most often comes out of a doctor's mouth when a patient asks about doing a low-carb diet for weight loss. The doctor issues a stern warning: "Your brain can't function properly unless you eat some number of carbohydrates three times daily, with more carbohydrate snacks in between." Big Food is happy to support and repeat this lie because the carbohydrates found in sugar and grains provide cheap ingredients that manufacturers can use to make all manner of tasty snacks.

It's obvious why Big Food is happy to repeat this lie, and most dietitians were trained in schools of nutrition founded and funded by Big Food. But why are doctors so quick to repeat it? We are taught the biochemistry of carbohydrate metabolism. We are taught that glucose (the sugar your body uses for energy) can be made from carbohydrates, proteins, and fats that we have eaten. Unfortunately, somewhere along the way doctors forget this training and buy in to the lie that humans must eat carbohydrates to function.

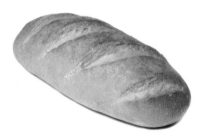

THE COMMON SENSE

There have been societies in which individuals lived their entire lives while eating a zero-carbohydrate diet for months at a time. These societies were well known to the scientific community in the past, and they should be well known to medical science as well. It seems that their good health and perfect dentition has currently been forgotten by both the scientific and medical communities.

For example, the Inuit tribes of the arctic regions of Alaska, Canada, and Greenland lived in a part of the world where few plants could grow. The majority of their diets (more than 90 percent by some estimates) was the fatty meat of whales, walrus, caribou, seal, and polar bears. It was so cold where they lived that it was impossible to grow plants. They would eat small amounts of berries, roots, and tubers during certain months of the year, but, on the whole, they ate very few, if any, carbohydrates for months at a time. Obviously, if the brain needed a certain amount of carbohydrates each day to function, the Inuit would have been extinct centuries ago. But they are still with us today despite the almost zero-carb diet, which was recorded by anthropologist Vilhjalmur Stefansson.

Stefansson lived among the Inuit for several years in the early twentieth century, and he was so impressed with the overall health of the people that he adopted their fatty-meat diet. When he returned to the United States and told of his dietary discovery, he was ridiculed and labeled as dishonest. To prove what he had witnessed, he agreed to be monitored for a full year of eating only meat. The skeptics watched closely as Stefansson flourished on his meat-only diet. He didn't develop any deficiencies, and he remained perfectly healthy.

Another community that flourished on a carnivore diet was the Masai people of Eastern Africa. The Masai diet was raw meat, raw milk, and raw blood from cattle. The tribe's dietary habits were studied closely by Dr. Weston A. Price, who reported that despite their zero-carbohydrate animal diet, they were very healthy and strong. Multiple other societies lived on meat almost exclusively, including the Cukotka in Russia, the Samburu and Rendille warriors of Africa, certain nomad tribes in Mongolia, the Sioux of South Dakota, and the gauchos from Brazil.

Today there are thousands of people who live very happily on zero-carb or very low-carb diets. They report being very healthy and energetic despite going for months at a time with no carbohydrates at all. There is no anthropological or physiological evidence that humans need to eat a certain amount of carbohydrates daily.

Some cells in the human body need glucose for energy. The red blood cells do not have a nucleus, or their own mitochondria, and thus they have no means of producing their own energy or burning fat as fuel. Certain cells in the brain and eye also need glucose for energy. However, your liver is perfectly capable of making all the glucose your body needs through a process called *gluconeogenesis*. Because the liver can produce as much glucose as these cells need to function perfectly, there is no need to eat carbohydrates.

THE RESEARCH

There is no meaningful research showing any need for daily carbohydrate intake in human beings. Although there are many "experts" who say otherwise, they don't have research to back up their claims. The liver can convert both amino acids and fatty acids into glucose for the cells that require glucose for fuel; you don't need to eat carbs.

THE TAKE-HOME

Many generations of humans have lived in situations where they had no access to carbohydrates for months at a time. Whether humans at one time did need carbohydrates and became genetically adapted to live without them or never needed them to start with is unknown, but at present you don't need to meet a minimum daily requirement for carbohydrates.

Most of the cells in your body can shift from needing carbohydrates as fuel to being able to burn some form of fat as fuel. Every human body has the biochemical machinery to make this shift from being a carbohydrate-burner to being a fat-burner; it just takes a little time to make the conversion. In no way does this limit your metabolic flexibility. Your body is always capable of burning carbs as fuel in the future, if you'd ever want that to happen.

For the few cells in your body that cannot use fat for fuel, your liver is happy to use gluconeogenesis to produce enough glucose to feed the cells just what they need. This process exists for a reason, and it clicks on without any effort on your part.

DO AS I DO

I often go days without eating anything but fatty meat cooked in either lard or butter. Some cuts of meat have 1 or 2 grams of carbohydrates, but that's not nearly the amount we are told we need to fuel our brains. I eat a little green veg now and then, but I do it more for taste than for the carbs. I have been low-carb or zero-carb for so long that my brain has adapted very well to burning fat as fuel, and my liver makes all the glucose my body needs for other functions on a moment's notice. Your body can do this, too.

HOMEWORK

Even though your doctor or dietitian might tell you your brain needs lots of carbs to function well, millions of people are doing great on a ketogenic diet. Here are two great resources to help you understand just what the body needs and what it does not.

BOOK: *Real Food Keto: Applying Nutritional Therapy to Your Low-Carb, High-Fat Diet* by Jimmy Moore and Christine Moore, NTP (2018)

This excellent resource helps you formulate an ancestrally appropriate ketogenic way of eating.

BOOK: *EAT RICH, LIVE LONG: MASTERING THE LOW-CARB AND KETO SPECTRUM FOR WEIGHT LOSS AND LONGEVITY* by Ivor Cummins and Jeffry Gerber, MD (2018)

Learn about the root causes of chronic disease and the diet that will prevent you from having them.

Chapter 23

GRILLING MEAT CAUSES CANCER

> **But it appears common, and has been found all over the world in all ages, that meat is considered the superior food, vegetables inferior or secondary.**
>
> —Vilhjalmur Stefansson

THE LIE

Eating charred meat cooked over an open flame will increase your risk of colon cancer or increase your risk of cancer overall.

WHY YOU SHOULD CARE

If grilling meat increases your risk of cancer then you should prepare the meat using another cooking method at a lower temperature. However, if grilling meat, as humans have done for thousands of years, does not increase your risk of cancer, then you can enjoy grilled meat without worry.

SUPPORT FOR THE LIE

This is another lie that has been virtually created by the World Health Organization (WHO) in one of their publications. There are several epidemiological observational studies that show a very weak correlation between grilled meat and risk for cancer. There are also a few rodent studies, most of which are poorly designed, that seem to show an increased risk of cancer in the rodent when it had been eating charred meat. However, the rodents in the studies consumed the supposed cancer-causing compounds at a level hundreds of times the amount the average human would eat.

There have been no randomized, controlled trials in humans that support this lie as being truth. Also, there are multiple observational studies that don't show any correlation between grilling meat and cancer risk. When you search for literature on this subject, it becomes obvious that there is much bias in the research, and the researchers have let emotional belief influence the conclusions of the study. Without blinding and/or randomization in their studies, this emotional bias seeps into the findings and undermines the research as reported.

THE COMMON SENSE

There is evidence that humans and our immediate predecessors have cooked meat over an open flame for hundreds of thousands of years, if not much longer. If there was any meaningful cancer risk from doing this, humans would either be extinct, or we would have stopped cooking meat by this method thousands of years ago. The trial-and-error of life tends to make an animal stop a certain behavior and pick up another behavior if there is a benefit in doing so. At some point in our history, we most certainly would have stopped grilling meat over an open flame if it yielded a cancer-causing meal.

The researchers on the WHO side of this argument are very emotionally invested in their viewpoint because they believe that a plant-based diet is best for humans and for the planet. Being so emotionally involved in such a research question makes the proponents of the grilled-meat-causes-cancer hypothesis very ardent and convincing. They are quick to promote their hypothesis as fact, even though it is barely a hypothesis. To the average observer, a passionate researcher seems very believable. However, being passionate and emotional about a topic does not make you correct.

THE RESEARCH

The WHO has proclaimed that certain compounds in grilled meat lead directly to cancer. They have based this opinion on the results of epidemiological observational research studies that seem to show a correlation between these compounds and cancer of various forms. Remember, though, that this type of research can show a correlation, but it can never *prove causation*. The studies show only the slightest correlation between eating grilled meat and cancer risk, and the relative risk is very low—almost nonexistent. The same style of studies were used to show the link between smoking and lung cancer, but with a big difference.

The studies on smoking and cancer showed a very high correlation with a very high relative risk. This means it is very, very likely that smoking increases lung cancer risk, even though the research doesn't prove the causation. The participants in the study had no other confounder in common that could explain the increased cancer incidence in the smokers.

The questionable compounds in grilled meat are acrylamides (ACs), heterocyclic amines (HCAs), and polycyclic aromatic hydrocarbons (PAHs). In rodent studies, these compounds from the grilled meat were highly correlated with cancer in mice and rats, but the quantities of the compounds were thousands of times the amount a human would ever eat. One problem with using the rodent studies to draw conclusions for humans is that humans have grilled meat over an open flame for hundreds of thousands of years, whereas rodents have not. Another issue is that rodents have a different diet than humans and a very different digestive system. There have been no randomized, controlled trials in humans, and there aren't even any observational studies that come close to showing a strong correlation, or causation, between eating grilled meats in normal amounts and increased cancer risk.

THE TAKE-HOME

Rats and mice in the wild eat berries, bugs, grain, and sometimes raw meat. They never eat grilled meat, and they never have. To feed them high levels of compounds produced by grilled meats is sure to upset their system because it is not their ancestral food. In the studies to determine a relationship between grilled meat and cancer, the rodents ate levels of these compounds thousands of times higher than even the most fervent human carnivore would eat. This obviously doesn't prove much.

Since before recorded history, humans have been grilling fresh meat over an open flame. It is part of our ancestral diet as far back as archeology and anthropology can track. If you've ever tried to cook fresh meat over an open flame, even with the most modern grilling equipment, you know the impossibility of not charring at least some of the meat. Thus, it defies common sense to claim that humans should be afraid of grilled meats, even when they eat grilled meats on a daily basis.

Two of the compounds in grilled meat that we're supposed to be afraid of, HCAs and PAHs, do cause increased incidence of cancer when consumed at thousands of times the normal levels. But that's the key information: *thousands of times the normal levels*. So, in other words, you shouldn't eat more than one hundred grilled rib-eye steaks daily. Obviously, though, that's way beyond what anyone is going to consume. Also, would it surprise you to hear that these compounds occur in many other foods the WHO considers very safe for you to eat? Well, they do.

ACs appear in some foods naturally, and they're in any fried food and any food that has been browned. French fries, toast, prune juice, breakfast cereals, roasted nuts, coffee, cocoa, potato chips, and cookies are examples of foods in which we can find ACs. When you toast bread until it is even a little brown, you create acrylamides, and those acrylamides are added to the acrylamides produced in the bread when it was baked.

Cooking vegetables causes high levels of a compound called benzopyrene, which is thought to increase cancer risk. (Why this is not talked about more is a subject for another day.) Any food that contains amino acids—the building blocks of protein, creatine, and sugar—can produce HCAs and PAHs. This includes any bread, veggies, and potatoes that have any meat juice on them at all. We know these vegetable-source foods contain proteins, because our vegan friends tell us so, and they definitely contain sugars because that is what carbohydrates are made from. If these plant foods come into contact with meat during their cooking, then they can produce HCAs and PAHs. To avoid HCAs and PAHs, you would have to eat all of your food in its raw form—no cooking allowed. Obviously, this is not what humans have been doing for thousands of years. We have been cooking at least some of our food since fire was harnessed as a tool, and it's very common to cook meat and plant foods together.

DO AS I DO

I have no fear of grilled meat. I eat it as often as I can, and I feed it to my family as often as I can. The research on this subject is trivial at best, and it's filled with researcher bias. Until meaningful research is produced that shows that the way our ancestors prepared their food is now dangerous, I will continue to enjoy it.

HOMEWORK

Grilling meat over an open flame is just about as human as you can get. Despite the many resources that perpetuate the myth and misconceptions, there are some reliable sources of information out there. Here is a great one.

BOOK: *THE BIG FAT SURPRISE: WHY BUTTER, MEAT & CHEESE BELONG IN A HEALTHY DIET* by Nina Teicholz (2014)

Teicholz destroys the silly arguments that meat is somehow unnatural and unhealthy for you.

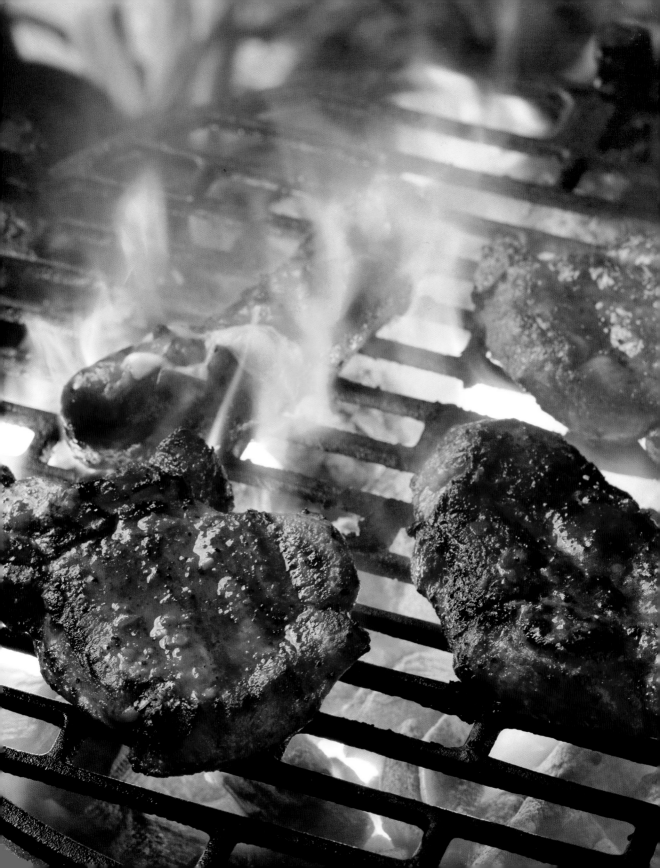

Chapter 24

EATING PROCESSED MEAT CAUSES CANCER

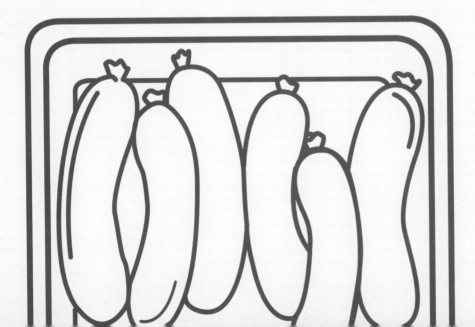

"

Beware of false knowledge; it is more dangerous than ignorance.

—George Bernard Shaw

"

THE LIE

Processed meats, such as bacon, sausage, bologna, and hot dogs, contain high levels of nitrates and nitrites which will cause you to have cancer.

WHY YOU SHOULD CARE

If processed meats are full of nitrates and nitrites, and these nitrates and nitrites increase your risk of cancer, then you should limit or avoid them. However, if processed meats contain fewer nitrates and nitrites than many vegetables, and these compounds have not been definitively shown to increase cancer risk, then you can enjoy processed meats as part of a healthy, affordable diet.

SUPPORT FOR THE LIE

The International Agency for Research on Cancer (IARC), an organization working under the World Health Organization (WHO), announced that processed meats were a probable cause of cancer. The group formed this opinion based on research from animal (rodent) studies, observational studies, and population studies. IARC claimed to have 800 studies showing the connection between processed meats and cancer, but fewer than five of these studies are published. These epidemiological studies show a very weak correlation between eating processed meats and increased cancer risk. At the time I'm writing, there have been no controlled trials that prove this hypothesis.

Nutritionists, dietitians, and many other experts accept as fact that processed meats are a cancer risk. The official consensus is that processed meat is dangerous, and we should avoid it. It is considered unacceptable, almost taboo, for a doctor or other health/nutrition professional to question this belief.

THE COMMON SENSE

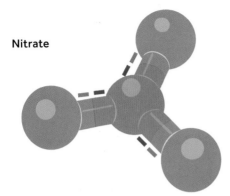

Nitrate

Nitrates are chemical ions containing a nitrogen atom and three oxygen atoms arranged as in the illustration above. Nitrates can occur naturally in soil, can be made by bacteria, or can be synthetically made. Nitrates occur at very high concentrations in celery and beets. Nitrates are currently being researched for their medicinal purposes, as they improve blood pressure and reduce the risk of heart attack.

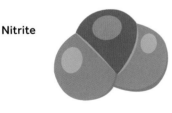

Nitrite

Nitrites are chemical ions containing a nitrogen atom and two oxygen atoms arranged as in the illustration above. Nitrites occur naturally, can be made by bacteria, can be synthetically made, and are produced in human saliva at hundreds of times the concentration found in cured meats. Nitrites also can be formed by chemically converting the nitrates found in celery and beets.

Processed meats do indeed contain nitrates and nitrites. The U.S. Department of Agriculture has set very strict guidelines on the amounts of nitrates and nitrites that can be in processed meats: Less than 500 parts per million can be used in the production process, and often only 10 parts per million remain in the finished product. This amount might seem worrisome until you hear how much nitrate and nitrite are in many other foods and in your saliva.

For example, many vegetables contain much higher levels of these ions than processed meat. Celery and beet greens contain hundreds of times more than the average hot dog. Somehow, those groups that warn us of the dangers of processed meats overlook this fact. Imagine if experts told us to avoid vegetables because of their water content but said it's perfectly safe for us to drink a glass of water. This makes no sense, and neither does the nitrate/nitrite scare.

More than 90 percent of the nitrates the average person consumes comes from vegetables. Yes, you read that right. Celery, beet greens, and arugula contain more nitrates than one hundred hot dogs! If we are worried about nitrates, and the compounds they produce, then we should strictly limit veggies rather than processed meat.

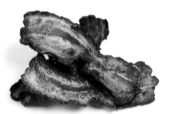

Here's some information you might find surprising: The bacon and hot dogs that say "uncured," "organic," and "nitrate-free" contain more nitrates than the cheaper processed meat and hot dogs. Apparently we're supposed to consider the nitrates in organic and nitrate-free meats to be different because they come from celery and beet juice. A loophole in U.S. federal guidelines makes it permissible to ignore this nitrate (which is the exact same molecule as the one used in cheaper processed meat). So if a company uses celery juice as the source of nitrates, it gets to call the meat product "nitrate-free," even though the final nitrate amount is much higher than in other products.

Would you be surprised to hear that more than 90 percent of the nitrites you swallow each day do not come from food at all but from your saliva? Well, it's true, and it really puts the final nail in this myth's coffin. Your body naturally produces hundreds of times more nitrites in your saliva each day than you could possibly get if you ate nothing but processed meat all day. Should we outlaw your spit as a possible carcinogen?

Hopefully, you're getting a sense of how foolish it is to be afraid of the small amount of nitrates and nitrites left in processed meats. If you truly fear nitrates then you should stop eating green vegetables. And if you fear nitrites then you should stop swallowing your own saliva.

THE RESEARCH

The research supporting this lie is laughable. When the paper from M.I.T. that started this scare was first published, the news media picked it up and ran with it. Lots of people heard the news. However, when the paper was later discredited and retracted, you barely heard a peep.

People who frequently eat processed meat tend to be less affluent than those who do not. They also tend to smoke more, exercise less, and do other unhealthy things. When researchers who performed the observational studies that show a correlation between processed meat and cancer risk were collecting their data, they used those untrustworthy Food Frequency Questionnaires (FFQs), and they did not take these confounding variables into account. They did not control for these other unhealthy behaviors, so the research is tainted. If someone who eats lots of hot dogs also smokes, drinks lots of beer, and never gets off the couch, are we surprised that their rate of having cancer is higher than someone who avoids hot dogs, doesn't smoke, works out, and drinks only rarely? I'm not. Were the hot dogs to blame? Almost certainly not. This obvious defect in the research is ignored by most experts who try to give us advice about the dangers of processed meat.

THE TAKE-HOME

This lie is another great example of a situation in which researcher bias and personal beliefs have been ensconced in nutrition dogma. When you look at the research with a critical eye, the lie completely falls apart. When you discover that "uncured" meat contains more nitrates than inexpensive processed meat, the situation becomes embarrassing. When you understand that your own saliva is by far the greatest source of nitrites in your body, the myth becomes completely laughable.

DO AS I DO

I enjoy processed meat as often as I like. I regularly feed my children hot dogs, bologna, and bacon. I have no fear whatsoever of the nitrates and nitrites in processed meats. I have, however, banned my family from eating vegetables and swallowing their own saliva. No, no—just kidding. But you get my point.

HOMEWORK

The following articles provide additional information about the nitrate and nitrite myth.

WEB ARTICLE: *"THE NITRATE AND NITRITE MYTH: ANOTHER REASON NOT TO FEAR BACON"* by Chris Kresser at http://bit.ly/DontFearBacon

Chris Kresser destroys the nitrate/nitrite myth and offers multiple references for more information in this great blog post.

WEB ARTICLE: *"DOES BANNING HOTDOGS AND BACON MAKE SENSE?"* by Sandy Szwarc, BSN, RN, CCP, at http://bit.ly/BaconIsGood

Sandy explains the silliness of worrying about the nitrites in processed meat if you ignore the nitrites in veggies, and she provides lots of great references you can research yourself.

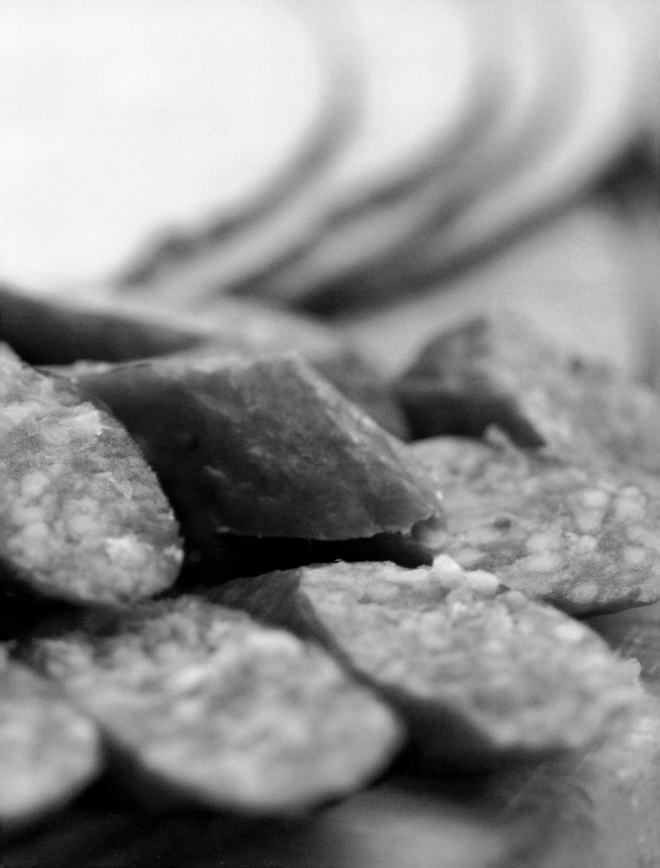

Chapter 25
LITTLE WHITE LIES

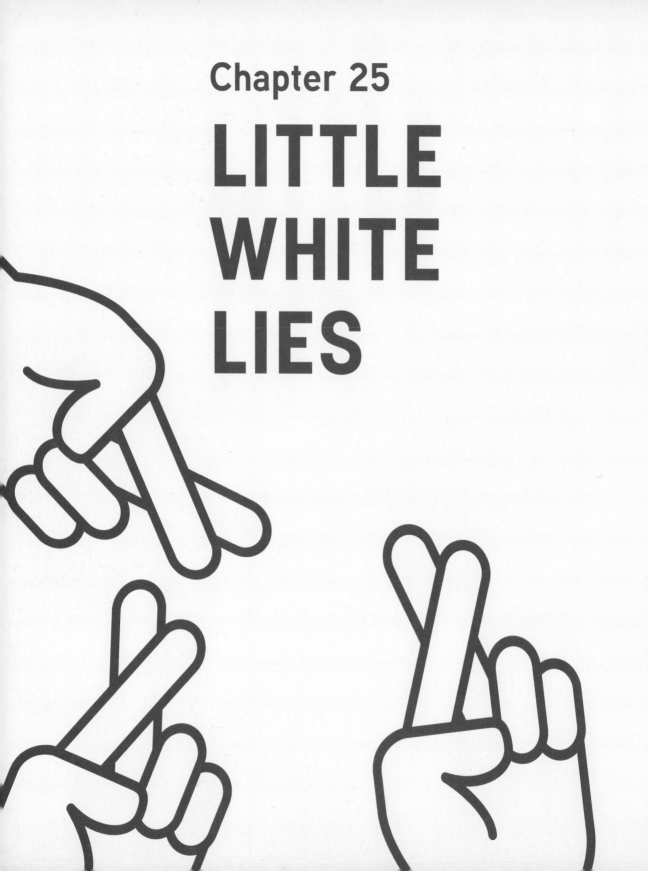

> ## Be careful about reading health books. You may die of a misprint.
>
> *—attributed to* Mark Twain

Various little white medical lies, like the ones in this chapter, are almost too numerous to count. I've included the most common ones here, along with a brief response to each. It's usually a relative or friend who tells you these lies, but there are still some doctors who also repeat them. If you hear one of these lies from your doctor, try to determine if he's joking. If he isn't, then run–don't walk– from his office in search of another source of medical care. Any doctor worth his co-pay should know better than to repeat any of these little white medical lies.

I've included these mostly for fun but also so you can tell the source of the lie that he or she is wrong. I'm a bit of a stickler over such things. We're supposed to be an intellectual, technologically advanced species. That should mean we don't believe silly things that aren't true. We should believe and repeat only things that are supported by evidence.

With that being said, here are some lies you can dispel for your friends and relatives.

We use only 10 percent of our brains.

MR (magnetic resonance) and PET (positron emission tomography) scans repeatedly have shown this statement to be false. To give this lie credibility, some people attribute it to Albert Einstein. All of your brain is working all the time— which is either a good thing or a bad thing, depending on how you use it.

You should drink at least eight glasses of water a day. Or more!

This lie likely comes from a recommendation the Nutrition Council made in the 1940s. That group recommended we ingest 64 ounces of fluids each day, but that recommendation was intended to include the water in the food we eat and in beverages other than water. No research has ever shown that you need a certain amount of clear water each day for health or weight loss. However, it's probably a good idea for you to drink a few glasses of good water every day. Your thirst mechanism is hard-wired, and it's very good at telling you how much fluid you need each day. It doesn't need your help in deciding how much water you should drink.

Shaved or cut hair grows back thicker and darker.

This lie has been disproved many times. I know; I know; it sure seems like the hair grows back darker and thicker, but it doesn't. I once argued with a cosmetologist about this lie and almost ended up exchanging blows over the topic. She assured me that this lie was definitely true, and her cosmetology textbook verified the statement. She said she would show me. Alas, after diligently searching for this lie in her book, without success, she decided to settle for throwing the book at me.

Reading in dim light (or watching TV too closely) is bad for your eyes.

Absolutely no research supports this lie. The human eye is one of the most impressive things in the known universe. Its ability to adjust to different situations is astounding. This lie was probably thought up by siblings who hated reading and wanted to mess with you. Or by your parent, who just wanted you to go outside to play.

Eating turkey will make you drowsy.

Turkey contains tryptophan, which is known to make you drowsy. The only problem with this little lie is that chicken, beef, and many other foods also contain as much (or more) tryptophan as turkey. What makes you drowsy (and fat) after a huge holiday meal are the starches and sugars, not the turkey.

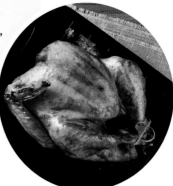

Don't let someone who's suffered a head injury fall asleep.
If your friend has been knocked out due to head trauma, a doctor should evaluate him. After he has been checked, your friend is perfectly safe to take a nap if he wants, even if he has a concussion. If a doctor tells you not to let your friend go to sleep after suffering a head injury, I want you to roll your eyes as far back in your head as possible, snap a selfie of you and that doctor, and send it to me. I might include it in my next book. Falling asleep presents no danger whatsoever to someone who has sustained a head injury. Indeed, doctors sometimes induce a coma in a patient with a severe head injury, causing them to sleep for days.

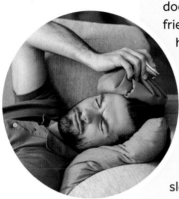

Swallowed chewing gum stays in your stomach or intestines for years.
Umm, no. I'm not sure when or where this lie started, but it has no basis in reality. The ingredients of chewing gum (a detailed list is quite hard to come by) are probably unhealthy, but gum can pass through the gut at the same speed as all the other foods you eat.

You should wait an hour after eating before you swim.
No research supports this lie. I used to enjoy making friends and relatives nervous at picnics with this one. I would eat a huge plate (or two) of food, announce immediately afterward that I was going for a swim, and then dive headfirst into the nearest body of water. The fact that I didn't cramp and die seemed to have no effect on the continued belief in this lie by my friends and family.

Fingernails and hair continue to grow after you die.
Not true. After a person dies, their skin dries out and contracts because they are no longer drinking their eight glasses of water per day. The skin pulls away from the nails, thus making the nails *appear* to grow. Dead things do not grow.

Spicy foods cause reflux, ulcers, or other stomach problems.

Some foods do inflame your stomach and intestines, but it's not the spicy foods you should worry about. Some spices can burn or tingle your tongue, but they don't affect your stomach or intestines. Your stomach constantly deals with concentrated hydrochloric acid and laughs at these wrongly accused spices. The more likely causes of stomach irritation are stress, medications, sugar, dairy, and grains. If your doctor suggests that you avoid spicy foods, again, roll your eyes *waaay* back and take a selfie for me to put on the cover of my next book.

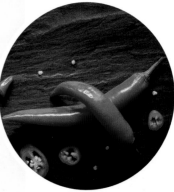

A woman can't get pregnant during her period.

Don't trust this one! Sperm can live in a woman's body for up to a week, and, as any woman can tell you, periods can be long or short, or even absent. It's unlikely that a woman will get pregnant from having sex during her true period, but it is definitely not 100 percent fail-safe.

You lose most of your body heat through your head.

According to research, probably done by scientists who were tired of being told by their moms to wear a hat when they go outside, you only lose 7 to 10 percent of your body heat through your head when you're outdoors in cold weather. Therefore, wear a hat if you want to, but it's optional. Feel free to tell your mom about this lie, but you should still wear your hat when you go out if she tells you to.

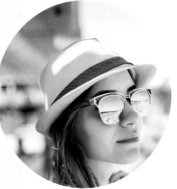

Suicide attempts increase over the holiday season.

Research shows that the suicide rate is lower during December than in other months. I am not sure how this lie got started. It was most likely started because it makes a good story. We are always eager to believe that there's a cause-and-effect relationship between things like the time of year or phase of the moon and some other unrelated occurrence. (See the myth related to the full moon later in this chapter.)

Poinsettias are deadly.

No confirmed human or animal death has occurred from eating poinsettias. Out of the thousands of episodes recorded by Poison Control of people or pets eating poinsettia, the worst symptoms ever reported were vomiting and stomach cramping, just as you experience when you eat any other nonedible plant. Poinsettias are not edible, and they don't taste good (yes, I tried a little piece while researching this book), but if you're thinking of poisoning your annoying uncle this Christmas season, the poinsettia is not the plant you will want to use.

Eating at night makes you fat.

The time of day you eat, according to the research, has nothing to do with weight gain. It's all about *what* you eat rather than when you eat it. No research supports this lie about eating at night—not even a little bit. Eat at whatever time of day you want; just make sure to eat the right foods.

Emergency room and labor and delivery visits increase during a full moon.

I realize I will offend many nurses (including my wife, a labor and delivery nurse) by saying that this lie has been studied and found to be false.

It's not even a little true. I discovered that this was a lie when I was an emergency room doctor and was planning to do a study about this relationship. At the time, I believed this statement to be true. I began to study and obtain data, but the numbers I collected from three different small-hospital emergency rooms weren't showing any relationship between trauma and the phase of the moon. After a little more research, I found out that the Mayo Clinic had already conducted a large study proving the phase of the moon was irrelevant to ER visits, and I abandoned my study. Sorry, nurses; please forgive me, but the truth must be known.

Coffee stunts the growth of children.

My grandmother was a firm believer in this lie. Therefore, I was forbidden to drink coffee until I was sixteen. Of course, I was sneaky and would drink coffee whenever I could without getting caught. I had an aunt who didn't believe this lie, and she had given all six of her children coffee without harming them. She used to sneak me some coffee when Granny wasn't looking. I have friends from Central America who tell me that coffee is an every-morning beverage for most children there; kids start drinking it when they're as young as three. Everyone there grows up just fine.

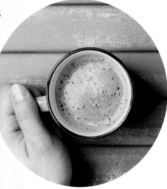

Apparently, this lie was started by C. W. Post (the cereal maker), who was trying to market his breakfast drink, Postum. His ad campaign warned American parents of the evils of coffee because he was trying to shame them into switching their child's morning drink from coffee to Postum, which was made from wheat and molasses. Postum was much less healthy for children than good old coffee.

Sugar intake makes kids hyper.

There is a long list of valid reasons why I encourage you to limit your child's sugar intake, but this isn't one of them. This lie sprang from a letter written by a doctor and published in a pediatrics journal. No existing research supports this lie, although a great many parents (including myself) seem to see a correlation between sugar consumption and bad behavior. I also don't recommend giving children sugar close to bedtime.

Blood is blue until it's exposed to air.

There are several versions of this lie, and all are untrue. Blood is always red. It's a brighter shade of red when it is carrying a full supply of oxygen (as it flows through your arteries), but it's still red when the oxygen has been used (as it flows through your veins). Blood appears blue in your veins because of the color of the vein walls.

Eating lots of carrots improves your night vision.

Raw carrots are fairly good for you, but no research supports the idea that eating carrots improves night vision. This rumor probably started as British propaganda during World War II to encourage citizens to eat root vegetables. Root crops eaten raw are full of fiber and good nutrition, but there is no evidence they improve your vision.

You are born with all the neurons in your brain that you'll ever have.

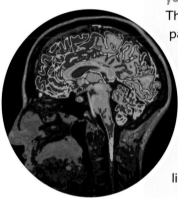

This terrible lie started long before we knew better. In the past, doctors, who had no research, believed that once you were grown, you could never form new neurons (nerve cells) in your brain. Good research has now proven that grown humans make new brain cells all the time. This is one of the reasons why eating a proper diet with plenty of healthy fats is good for your memory and lowers your risk of dementia. Your brain needs good nutrients to make new neurons. Some older doctors still believe this lie, but it has been completely disproved.

Ecstasy, meth, and some other drugs make holes in your brain.

Although these illegal drugs can have disastrous and permanent effects on brain function, none cause actual holes to form in the brain. I bet that this lie scares some kids into not trying drugs. However, you always should think about what might happen when your kids find out you lied to them. It is better to tell them the truth because it is as scary as the lie.

Brown sugar is better for you than white sugar.

I imagine this lie probably started because it resembles the stories that brown bread is better for you than white bread (a lie) and that brown rice is better for you than white rice (also a lie). Saying that brown sugar is better than white sugar is like saying unprocessed, organic poison is somehow better for you than processed poison. No, dummy; they're both poison.

Stretching before exercising prevents injury.

Every high school football coach in the world believes this lie is true, but it's not. Several studies have shown that stretching before physical activity doesn't decrease injury risk. It is, in fact, a waste of time. However, it does give football players something to do until the game starts.

Eating six small meals a day is ideal for managing diabetes or weight loss.

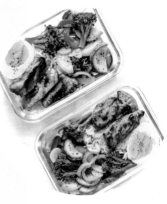

As with all the other lies, there is no research to back up this claim. Just like the *three square meals* advice of the past had no basis in research or medical fact, the idea of six small meals a day didn't have any scientific backing. You should eat as many times a day as you are hungry, whether this is once or four times. Eating six meals daily will keep your insulin level elevated and probably lead to weight gain. It's likely that you'll only get hungry six times per day if you're eating a high-carb, low-fat diet. Eating a diet with healthy fats produces a lasting sense of fullness, and you won't be hungry that often. Also, there is increasing research that shows that intermittent fasting (eating fewer meals each day) might be a much better strategy for long-term, meaningful weight loss.

Eating more protein makes muscles grow.

Protein doesn't make muscles grow unless you also are working out hard. Proteins are the building blocks of muscle tissue, but you must work those muscles to have muscle growth. Gorging on proteins does nothing but make your kidneys work hard to excrete the surplus protein and elevate your insulin level. Unless you engage in resistance exercise, protein won't make your muscles grow.

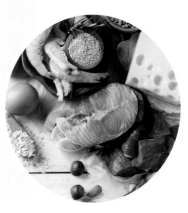

Cracking/popping your knuckles will lead to hand/finger arthritis.

Multiple studies show this lie to be false. Popping your knuckles causes no damage to your joints; therefore, it doesn't lead to long-term problems. However, if someone in your life is annoyed by the sound of knuckle-cracking, please be considerate and lay off the snaps, crackles, and pops in that person's presence.

Do you have a little medical white lie that your doctor or someone else has told you? Send it to me at **LMDTM@theberryclinic.com**, and I might use it in my next book.

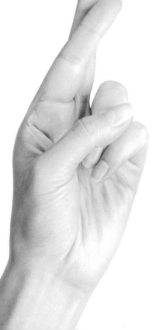

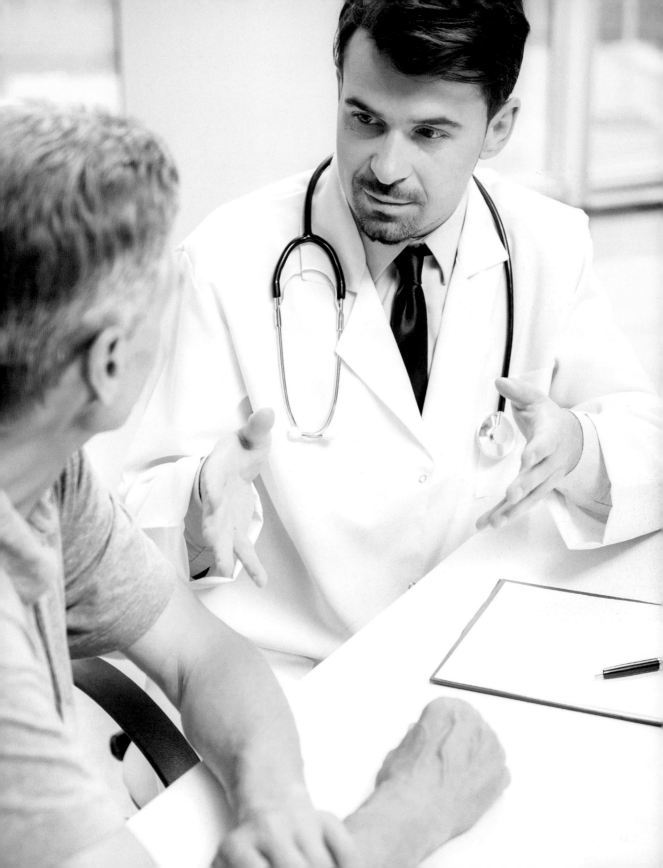

Chapter 26

DO AS I SAY, AND DO AS I DO

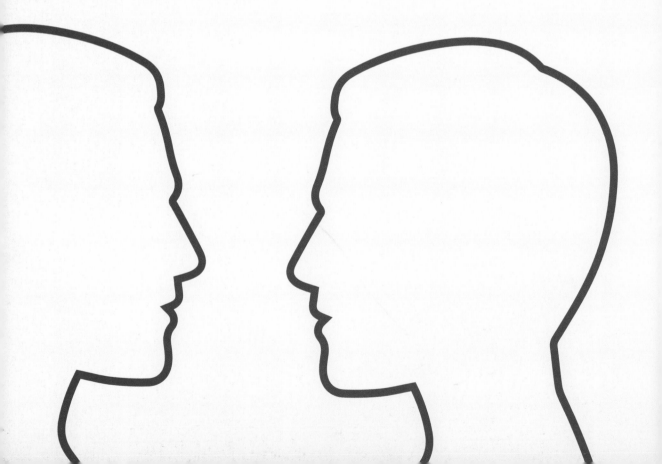

You have a cough? Go home tonight, eat a whole box of Ex-Lax—tomorrow you'll be afraid to cough.

—Pearl Williams

We've all heard some variation of the story of the preacher who told his congregation to follow the straight and narrow or face hellfire and damnation. When confronted with the fact he was often seen in the bar drinking and smoking and flirting with women, he frowned and said, "You should do as I say, not as I do!"

Many doctors live and act just like this preacher, and it's disappointing. Some doctors use tobacco while telling you not to, and others are quite obese but still feel they have the right to tell you how to lose weight. Many doctors are unhealthy and unhappy, but they don't think twice about preaching to you about how to be healthy and happy. If your doctor doesn't put his health first, even though he possesses all the knowledge he supposedly does, then why should you listen to him? This is one of the greatest embarrassing questions of modern medicine. How can a doctor have any credibility at all if he does the very things he tells you not to do? Perhaps state medical boards should focus more on this type of bad behavior than on some behaviors they currently give lots of attention.

As I mentioned earlier, one day in 2008, I realized I was a fat, unhappy, and unhealthy doctor who spent five days of his week *teaching* patients to lose weight and be healthy. These unpleasant conditions had crept up on me slowly. I was busy with my family, practice, and community, and I gave little thought to my health and what kind of impression I was making on my patients. I was a former high school athlete who had become so fat I couldn't breathe while tying my shoes. I obviously had to do something. I had always been an athlete, so I decided I'd start jogging on the treadmill to get back into shape. I kept eating pretty much as I had been (which is to say I kept eating terribly), but I figured I'd burn off any extra calories with the increased exercise. My plan was to burn more calories than I ingested. Of course, in medical school I had learned that this type of calorie deficit should guarantee weight loss.

I started my new regimen and was doing pretty well in the exercise department, but after a month I had gained a pound instead of losing. That was the last straw. Even though no other doctor in my community seemed interested, I had always suspected there was more to nutrition than I had learned in medical school. I was beginning to believe the answer to my weight problem might somehow be connected to this deficiency in knowledge. So, like a good student, I hit the books.

I read a couple of the popular low-fat diet books and wasn't impressed. I then read *The South Beach Diet* and *The Atkins Diet.* They both seemed to make more sense than the low-fat diet books. I kept looking and eventually came across two other books: *The Primal Blueprint* and *The Paleo Diet.* These books were

> 66
>
> **I realized I was a fat, unhappy, and unhealthy doctor who spent five days of his week *teaching* patients to lose weight and be healthy.**

about both diet and lifestyle, and they made an incredible amount of sense. I capped off my reading with two more books about the Paleo/Primal diet, spent hours reading research studies on PubMed, and read several other books that seemed to be on the right track. The key concepts I came up with were not new. In fact, they were as old as the human species itself. These ideas were so old and seemingly forgotten that we were having to rediscover them. To many people, they seemed to be new, or even faddish, ideas.

I can summarize the concepts with these statements:

- We humans have been on this planet an incredibly long time.

- For 99.99 percent of that time, we never, ever ingested grains, sugar, or milk; we never drank fruit juices or high-calorie liquids.

- We lived mostly on fatty meat and green plants, seeming to prefer the fatty meat when we could catch it.

- To get the health, mind, and body we want, we must honor our past way of eating and living and realize that our DNA hasn't had time to catch up with all the starches, sugars, and grains we are taught to consume in our modern life.

- Your DNA responds to unnecessary sugars and starches by putting them right where you don't want them as adipose tissue on your belly, butt, and thighs.

- Your body also puts this adipose tissue in your liver, where it can lead to abnormal liver function and severe liver disease.

To achieve the health you want and the body and mind you desire, you have to honor certain things. The following sections describe some of those things.

HONOR YOUR HUMAN DNA

The DNA in your cells right now is the end product of more than 70,000 pairs of your ancestors reproducing successfully over eons of time. It should be difficult for you to think of yourself as a loser if you keep this fact in mind.

The DNA you've received from all those successful ancestors knows how to take care of itself; it likes certain things, it needs certain things, and it has no idea what to do with other things in your diet. Your DNA has become very good at working with and benefiting from your gut bacteria. Mutilating or mutating your bacteria with unnecessary antibiotics can have disastrous consequences on your health and your level of obesity. Your DNA needs certain nutrients to repair the cells and tissues of your body; otherwise, it can't optimize your body and your health.

Think about what your ancestors ate. That is what your DNA craves and what it knows how to use. Three major things your DNA has been exposed to only for the last few hundred years are grains, sugars, and the milk of another species. Most people across the world cannot drink milk without experiencing serious stomach upset. Their DNA doesn't code for the enzyme that breaks down the lactose in milk. Those of us who seem to be able to comfortably drink milk suffer more slowly and subtly from drinking it.

Feed your DNA what it has been eating the longest, and it will reward you with great physical and mental health. Your DNA and the parts of it that get turned on and off decide whether you will be healthy or not.

HONOR YOUR DIET

Your diet is the part of your environmental exposure that you have the most control over. You could organically grow every morsel of food that passes through your lips if you have the time, and you want to put effort into that endeavor. Because most of us are busy with other things, being organic farmers isn't usually an option. So, you have to do the best you can with the food you purchase and remember that you are literally made of what you eat. What you eat and drink becomes *you*, and the old computer idiom of garbage in, garbage out (GIGO) is a good way to think of your diet. Not every bit of food you ingest will be pristine and organic. However, if you do the best you can to fill your belly with natural whole foods, your health and your life will benefit.

HONOR YOUR ENVIRONMENT

The environment you live in is filled with things you allow into it, and it's void of the things you keep out. Therefore, if you fill your environment with tobacco smoke, junk food, and lots of stress, don't be surprised if you lead a shortened and miserable life. Avoiding toxins such as tobacco smoke, unsafe water, and unsafe food additives are simple things you can do to protect your environment. It's important that you avoid BPA (bisphenol-A), which is in certain food and beverage containers. When you heat a container of food or beverage that has BPA in it, the BPA leaches into the food and drink, and it can cause problems with your glands and hormones. This is just one example of the many things harming your environment that you might not have heard about or that you've not given much thought to. Of course, you can't control every substance in your environment because there are just too many. But when you put effort into honoring your environment, you will be rewarded with better mental and physical health.

HONOR YOUR ACTIVITY

Although it's not a great method for losing weight, daily exercise is very good for your body and mind in many other ways. Studies have shown that being active benefits you both physically and mentally. When you go to the store, don't drive around for five minutes looking for the closest parking space. Park at the end of the lot and walk. Most of the time you'll get in and out of the store more quickly by doing this. You'll also save gas and keep your mind and body in better shape. You can use little tricks like this to make your life a more active one without expending much effort or spending much money. Our ancestors walked a few miles each day, and sometimes they had to run very fast or lift heavy things. By making small efforts to do more of these activities in your modern life, you will replicate the lifestyle your DNA was accustomed to for thousands of years, and it will reward you for that. Don't waste time and money joining the gym unless you really love it and you have fun when you go there.

HONOR YOUR LAB WORK

After a certain age, you're wise to partner with an understanding, knowledgeable doctor and check meaningful lab values a few times each year. There are organs and systems in the human body that can start having subtle problems, and those problems worsen over years without causing any noticeable symptoms. Only with routine lab work can you and your doctor detect these problems early and correct them before you experience permanent damage. Many of the preventative tests recommended by the authorities serve little functional purpose; therefore, you must have a doctor you trust to guide you through the maze of medical testing options.

HONOR YOUR NEED FOR SCREENING

Early detection of diseases such as cancer greatly increases the chances that your doctor will be able to treat and cure them. Regular consultation with a trusted doctor leads to meaningful screening tests that identify early signs of cancer and other disease. Without a doubt, some screening tests are overused, misused, or both, but the wise use of screening tests by a competent doctor can increase both your health span and your life span.

HONOR YOUR TELOMERES

Telomeres are little areas of DNA at the end of your chromosomes, and it appears that they protect your DNA from damage and quite possibly help keep you from aging more quickly than necessary. Studies show that avoiding things like smoking, processed foods, toxic chemicals, and bad stress helps keep your telomeres from shortening prematurely, which slows aging and keeps you healthier and more energetic. The study of telomeres and ways to optimize them is an exciting branch of medical research right now, and new developments in this area should yield significant health benefits for you.

HONOR YOUR MITOCHONDRIA

These little powerhouses inside your cells provide the energy that your cells need to perform their best. You have to feed your mitochondria the correct diet and protect them from toxins; otherwise, they will become weak and sick, and they'll start to dwindle in number. Protecting your mitochondria is yet another reason to avoid toxins in what you breathe, eat, and drink. Your mitochondria are your best friends if you want to stay active and vigorous into older age. Therefore, you should treat them right. Research into how to optimize mitochondria is another exciting branch of medical research that should uncover some benefits for your health.

HONOR YOUR STRESS AMOUNT AND TYPE

We all experience both good stress and bad stress. Good stress is beneficial to your body and mind; it comes from things like challenging yourself with difficult games, puzzles, and sports; learning new things; and going new places. Bad stress is harmful to your health, and you should minimize your exposure to it as much as possible. Bad stress comes from things like bad relationships, a job you hate, a sedentary lifestyle, or negative thinking. Although these things might seem trivial, it's important that you be mindful of these things and continually make your life a place you enjoy living.

HONOR YOUR GUT BACTERIA

You might think of your body as a single entity, but it's more than that. The medical community is becoming increasingly aware that your body is an orchestra of many players—both human and non-human. New research, for instance, is showing that the trillions of bacteria living in your intestines are vital to the quality of your overall health. Those mitochondria I discussed earlier were almost certainly bacteria we lived with harmoniously for so long that we invited them to move in permanently. Focusing all your effort and resources on something like joining the gym or taking expensive supplements is folly; those things will never lead to the long-term improvements in your health that you desire. Only when you honor all of the things I've listed will you achieve and maintain the mental and physical health you want and deserve.

HONOR YOUR SLEEP

We sleep for one-third of our live. Although that may seem like a waste of time at first glance, good-quality sleep is intimately related to every facet of our health—both physical and mental. Protect your sleep environment like you would protect any treasure, and let nothing intrude.

Ensure your bedroom is as dark as possible. It should be cool and comfortable. Consider having only red light on in your bedroom after dark; alternatively, you could wear blue-blocking glasses. Only engage is pleasurable activities in your bedroom; never work, argue, or discuss difficult topics there. Have some form of white- or pink-noise source, so you are not awakened by bumps in the night. During sleep is the only time your brain activates the glymphatic system, which cleans, repairs, and renews your brain. Honor your sleep and protect your sleep environment.

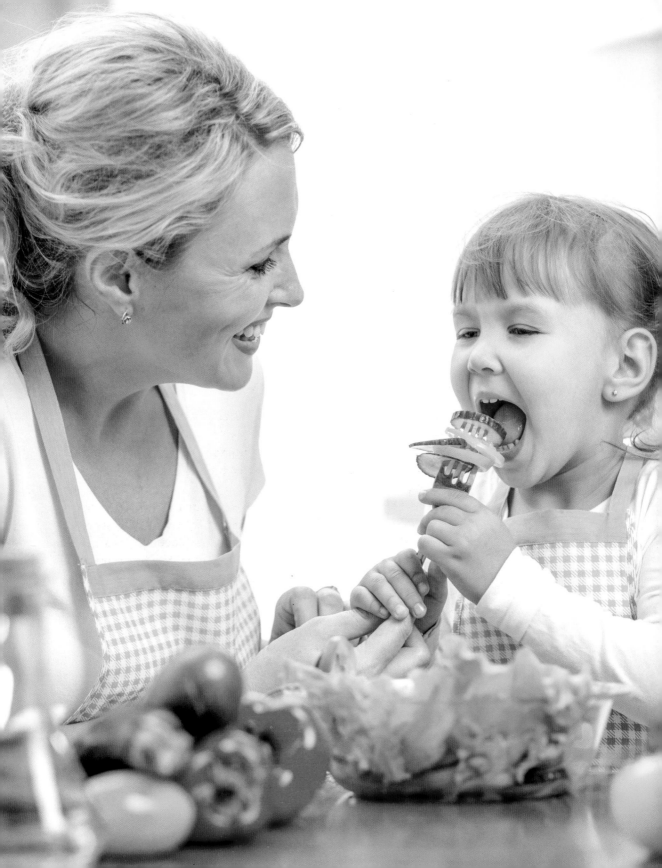

Chapter 27
DEAREST COLLEAGUES

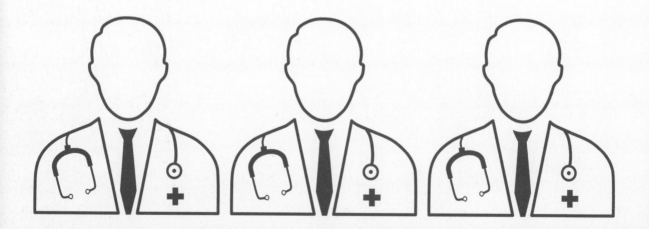

> **Doctors always think anybody doing something they aren't is a quack; also they think all patients are idiots.**
>
> —Flannery O'Connor

Shame on you. There was a time when almost everyone greatly trusted doctors. There was a time when doctors worked diligently to ascertain the truth for their patients, even if the truth wasn't what the patient wanted to hear. Doctors used to deliver bad news with the same discipline and character that they delivered good news. But some disturbing things have happened along the way. Doctors have become distracted and disenchanted, stopped paying attention, and—worse—stopped caring. Some of us have slowly morphed from healers and teachers into corporate medicine zombies and Big Pharma pill-pushers. I know this because I went down this road for a few years. I used to caution patients with diverticulosis about eating seeds and nuts, and I warned all patients to stay out of the sun. I used to tell patients to cut back on salt, and I wrote many high-dose statin prescriptions in my early career. But remember, dear colleague: We don't *do* medicine. We *practice* medicine. This means we are supposed to improve as the years pass. Are you improving in the advice and counsel you give your patients each year? (Hint: Knowing lots of details about the newest, expensive Big Pharma pill is not a sign of getting better at practicing medicine.)

> **There is often so much politics in medicine that being right can actually get you into trouble.**

There is redemption and forgiveness in every good story as long as it's deserved and earned. Your patients look up to you blindly and trustingly. They follow your advice in the face of facts and friends telling them to do otherwise. They are potentially harmed by your pills and your procedures, as well as by your indifference to the truth and your push for profit. You are well aware of your frustration, laziness, and ennui. The earned pride that you once felt and the deserving self-respect you once enjoyed are withering and crumbling.

You hate the style of unthinking medicine you're practicing, and the patients don't like it either. They are being awakened by thoughtful, articulate experts in other fields of health, from herbal medicine to acupuncture. The Internet has given your patients access to more meaningful medical research and knowledge than ever before. Patients now have more medical research at their fingertips than the best of doctors used to have. Despite how you might feel about that situation, it's a very good thing. If you found yourself with a case of cognitive dissonance from reading that last statement—or if you get upset when your patient brings printed info from a website when they visit you—then you have a problem. If you don't start righting past wrongs, there will soon come a day when you and your profession will be no more respected than politicians or used-car salesmen. You will lose your title of expert and healer, and you will be looked upon as pretentious and usually wrong. There are people who have no special training who post videos on YouTube that give better advice on nutrition and weight loss than you currently do. Every day, new videos are posted by people from all walks of life who have a greater grasp of nutrition, prevention, and how to apply both to real human problems than you do. If that last statement riles you up, then good. I want to piss you off, slap you around, and wake you up before you ruin the practice of medicine for all of us.

You are losing credibility. Patients once had only their doctor to go to with questions about their health and only their doctor to trust. There was no Internet, and the average town's library shelves had only a few dusty old medical books and journals. If a patient didn't believe the doctor, the person's only choice was to see another doctor, who usually was in another town. The odds were likely that the patient would hear the same verdict from the second doctor, and the matter was then settled. Only those with financial means could travel to larger facilities and specialists. Once there, they might receive better news or a different plan of care, but that wasn't always the case. Doctors didn't know everything back then either, but there was no way for patients to fact-check them.

Today it is different. Your patients can check the validity of your diagnosis on a website on their cell phones as they sit in your exam room. You might not have even finished your sentence yet. Your patients can consult experts from around the world via Skype and other services, and they can watch videos on the way to and from your office. Upon arriving home, patients can know just as much about their diagnosis as you do, and they might even discover that you don't know what you're talking about.

In this environment of increased information availability, we doctors find ourselves in both the scariest and the most exciting time to practice medicine. Merely wearing the white coat and draping the stethoscope over your shoulders will not save you from the world of near-instant information your patients can access. If you thought you would comfortably cruise through your career in medicine, and no one would ever discover you had become intellectually lazy or had stopped caring, you were wrong. If you hope to remain respected and relevant, then you must read broadly and deeply, not only in your specialty and in your field but also in other fields. You can rest assured that your patient is reading opinions of their symptoms and conditions from experts in multiple disciplines because the information is supremely important to them. Understand this: Your patients don't care where they get good nutrition and wellness advice; they're just as happy to get it from the Internet as from you. If you're not willing to discuss their Internet research with them, distill it, add to it, and ultimately synthesize a working diagnosis with them, you will become as obsolete as a VCR player and as disrespected as an exposed charlatan. If, however, you choose to step up to this challenge, you will enjoy relationships of mutual respect with your patients that your predecessors would have only dreamed of. You will become a trusted and loved adviser, expert, and friend.

It's not too late. No matter how far you've allowed yourself to drift into frustration, laziness, and blind belief in what the American Academy of Whatever and the latest Big Pharma company-sponsored research tells you, you can turn your career around and move slowly but surely back to the rewarding and awesome career of being a doctor. If you're a specialist, don't fall blindly for the latest procedure, no matter how great the remuneration. If meaningful research doesn't show improved long-term outcomes from the new procedure, then don't perform it. If you're a primary care physician, don't fall for the catchy spiel of a smooth-talking drug rep without fact-checking the story for yourself. If you fail to do this, your patient's health and your reputation will suffer. You might be protected from professional sanctions by following the latest guidelines, but you will not be protected from the disgust and disenchantment your patients feel for you if the guidelines are later revealed to be folly. You may only remember your patients as a blur of humanity. Your patients remember you quite clearly as the doctor who either got it right or got it wrong.

Be very careful about repeating anything to your patients as medical fact if it hasn't been proven. Once a medical lie takes hold, it can take decades to remove it from our collective memory. An example is the lie that testosterone replacement will cause prostate cancer. This lie, as you may know, began in the 1940s because of the belief of one respected and credible doctor. The misinformation quickly spread to the brains of all learned professors and teachers in the profession. They promptly passed the lie on to all their medical students (including you), who in turn spread it to the world as they began to practice. The fallacy quickly spread to the news media, who shared the information with everyone with a television or a magazine subscription. Most experts in urology now know that testosterone does *not* cause prostate cancer. However, a great many doctors, patients, and patients' families still believe it to be true. The quality of patients' lives and relationships are being negatively affected because of this sort of medical lie. Please verify that the advice you give your patients has been distilled through both common sense and meaningful research.

ADVICE FOR MEDICAL STUDENTS

M1 to M4: You've made it to medical school. Now, if you only had more hours in the day! I can remember sitting in my tiny library study room and thinking that if I took even a one-hour nap, it could lead to failure in pharmacology class. I feel your pain, but don't lose hope. Reading lots of research on various topics is not something you have time for yet. So, I want to share a few tips that will give you a much better chance of having a happy, successful practice when you get to that point. If you can ingest these few nuggets of knowledge and apply them to your present and future life, I think you will be a better doctor for it.

First, we are not even close to knowing everything there is to know about medicine, the body, and the mind. As you sit in your classes, you can get the impression that all has been discovered and written down about a given subject and that your professor plans to test you about all of it on the next exam. You do need to pay attention and do well in your classes, but you also need to remember your professors are human, fallible, and very proud of their positions in life. You just want to do well on your exams and get through this period with the best medical education possible. When you combine all the facts in the last two sentences and add lots of insecurities, fears, pressures, and dreams to the mix, you have a training plan that can lead you to being much less of a doctor than you could have been otherwise.

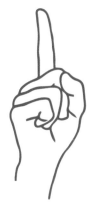

Helping people live the happiest and healthiest lives they can is an amazing career. Trust me; you want to be very good at it. By remembering a few key concepts now, you will be preparing yourself for success later.

Leeches were once standard of care. I say this to remind you never to forget that things you're taught are brilliant ideas today might be stupid tomorrow. The best doctors in the country once proudly used leeches to treat many diagnoses; leeches were the *standard of care.* If a doctor at that time had told other doctors who were using leeches it was stupid and dangerous, they would have run him out of town. Just because the American Academy of Whatever recommends doing or not doing something does not give you the leisure of leaving your thinking cap at home. You're responsible for your patients' health and helping them to prevent disease. The various guidelines are often published to stoke egos or plump up Big Pharma bank accounts. Sometimes standing up against something you think is wrong is scary and takes quite a bit of courage, but you went into medicine to be a hero and make a positive difference in your patients' lives, right?

Your professors are not gods, but don't argue with them in class. Lecture halls and medical journals are designed to appear as if the information they contain came down from on high. Your professor and clinical instructors are human, and they make mistakes. They're trying their best, but they might very well be repeating a medical lie to you as part of your education. Be alert for these lies, but don't point it out if you think you hear one. Overall, teachers don't appreciate being called out for being wrong, especially in front of the whole class. You are very busy and have little time for extra-curricular study, so if an instructor teaches you something that seems to go against common sense or the research as you currently understand it, file it away and research it more thoroughly when you get a chance.

Read the entire study, not just the conclusion. If you've ever seen a news report about a medical subject and thought the point the reporter was trying to make was silly, then you know what can come from reading only the conclusion of a medical study and then acting on it. Conclusions are in articles to save time for the reader—not for people to use to make medical treatment decisions. As you begin to read medical studies, pay careful attention to how often the conclusion doesn't follow from the findings or how the study design is flawed enough to give questionable results.

Always be looking for inconsistencies, but ask about them respectfully. Any time something said in lecture doesn't make sense to you or seems backward to your way of thinking, remember it. You might not have time to research it right now, but you will find the time later. Learned scholars behave this way. You should never blindly, dumbly accept what you are told, no matter how long the lecturer's white coat is. Look for inconsistencies now, but point them out later. Remember—you're trying to become a thoughtful, intelligent medical professional rather than an apostle who blindly follows a medical dogma.

You have a responsibility to know what you're talking about. When you become a doctor, you will be responsible for the professional advice you give your patients, and you're accountable for the outcome of bad advice. Make sure that your medical opinions and logic are rock-solid. You shouldn't just repeat what you've been taught; you should dispense advice based on what you have thought and what you have learned. There is a difference.

ADVICE FOR NEW DOCTORS

M-5 to M-9: If you're fresh out of med school, you have big ideas and big dreams for your future. As you're busy with your residency duties, or just finishing up, your present duties and future obligations take up almost your every waking minute. You've been in the game long enough to know that some attending physicians are very good at being doctors, whereas others are full of crap. You have to make it your mission not to become an attending physician who is full of crap. Let me give you a few suggestions to help you wind through this medical maze.

You have to look like you know what you're talking about but also always be doubting what you think you know. "Read or perish, reread or suffer," was the advice given to me early in my career by a respected mentor. There is a very fine line between exuding the confidence patients need to see in you to trust you, and in being a sophomoric, arrogant know-it-all. Walking this thin line will be part of your daily duty for the rest of your career. Doctors who are self-doubting in front of patients inspire no confidence, and doctors who act like they know it all, even when they don't, are dangerous. Be neither.

Patients don't esteem doctors for their actual ability because they can't truly know your ability; it's their perception of your ability that matters. Some of the worst doctors I ever worked with were held in God-like reverence by their patients. Conversely, some of the smartest doctors I've known didn't inspire confidence in their patients because those doctors weren't self-confident. Your goal should be to carry the perfect blend of public confidence and private self-doubt. This will make it easier for your patients to believe in you while at the same time enabling you to keep your clinical acumen sharp and ready. You owe it to yourself and your patients to keep reading, studying, and thinking.

Keep reading! I can't emphasize this point strongly enough. You must keep reading and learning; otherwise, your body of available knowledge, and the depth of your differential diagnosis, will shrivel over the years. Most of us have been around an older doctor who had neglected his reading for so long that he recognized only ten different diagnoses and prescribed the same five medicines. Don't be that doctor.

Read outside your specialty. It goes without saying that you need to stay current in your field, but your responsibility goes much further than that. Some of the most rewarding cases I've cracked came about because of something I had read about that was totally outside my specialty. To be truly helpful to your patients, you have to know a lot about a lot, whether you are a primary care physician or a specialist.

Read outside the field of medicine. Be an eager student with an unquenchable thirst for knowledge in all areas of life. There is an intellectual strength that comes from being widely and deeply read. Often, the only way to synthesize a difficult diagnosis is with knowledge from several sources, and the key is sometimes knowledge you find outside the field of medicine. Remember, humans and their health are not separate from the rest of the world; they are right in the middle of it.

Shut up and listen to your patients, and they will tell you their diagnosis 90 percent of the time. I once heard a doctor tell a patient to stop talking so he could examine her and diagnose her condition. I was stunned by the ignorance of this statement. I thought he was joking at first, but he was not. You need to keep your physical exam skills honed, but make no mistake: Your most valuable tools are asking questions and listening to answers. The history you glean from listening to your patient is the key to diagnosis. Never forget that.

You will have hard days; suck it up. It's true that the doctor doesn't get to be sick. The doctor also doesn't get to be wrong. The buck stops with you, and it always will. You are ultimately responsible for every single thing that is done under your name and written above your signature. This is all the more reason to fill your head with knowledge and a differential diagnosis list as deep as the ocean.

ADVICE FOR YOUNGER DOCTORS

M-10 to M-15: Early in your practice, you have one million different things competing for your attention. You've made it through your training, and now you're trying to get the hang of being the doctor for your patients. Your practice is probably growing so quickly that you don't have much time to think of anything else. You squeeze in as much family and friend time as you can, but it's not enough. Let me share a few thoughts that might help you keep your head straight through this hectic time.

Keep reading! This is not optional. You have to stay abreast of the latest meaningful medical research. You can never lazily trust your patients' health to the opinion of older colleagues without verifying their recommendations against the research. Older doctors you will work with are often *right,* even when they're wrong. I was very bad at learning this lesson. You don't have to correct anyone else's paradigm; you are responsible only for yours. You have to show deference to older, respected doctors, even if they are wrong. Give them the respect they expect, while also protecting your patient from the doctor's error. You don't have to publicly point out when an older colleague is wrong; you just have to make sure his error doesn't affect your patient's care. If you are not actively reading and thinking, you are slowly falling behind, and so is the treatment your patients are getting from you.

Be a leader in your medical community. The competition is gaining on you. Herbalists, chiropractors, naturopaths, and other alternative practitioners are gaining your patients' trust. The public is trusting these alternative practitioners more and doctors less. By reaching out to these practitioners and building a working relationship with them, you continue to lead your patients' medical care. Many a doctor has bluffed and blustered when asked by a patient about some alternative therapy, only to have that patient never return to their clinic again. You no longer have the liberty of pretending everyone else is wrong and you are right. Join with other practitioners and lead them, or be left behind.

Build and solidify your practice financially. You will be much more likely to make medical decisions based on how they will affect your income if your finances are tight. Don't be the doctor who orders a CBC on every single patient you see because you are trying to pay off your CBC-machine. Work to become independent both financially and clinically so your treatment decisions for your patients remain pure and unbiased.

ADVICE FOR OLDER DOCTORS

M-15+: You have had some degree of success in your medical practice. Over the years, you have come to feel that you can handle anything a patient might bring to you. Usually, after just a few words from a patient, you already know their diagnosis and what treatment they need. However, you then have to sit politely and let them finish their story before you can talk about their diagnosis and treatment plan. You have to remind yourself that sometimes hoofbeats are from a zebra because you now know how rare zebras are. This is a very dangerous time in your practice for you and for your patients.

If your career as a student is over, then your career as a doctor should be over as well. The reason I love the M numbering system is that it reminds me that I am still a student. (As I write this, I'm an M-21.) I am still learning—not just details, but whole new paradigms concerning medicine, nutrition, and health. Reading and rereading are just as important for you now, my dear colleague, as they were when you were a lowly M-1. If you think you know everything there is to know, or even if you think you know all you need to know, you are a danger to every patient you treat. It's so easy to become complacent (lazy), jaded (bored), and burned out (done) that you can't bring yourself to question long-held truths and newly published ones. Well, tough. You chose to wear a title that means *teacher*, and you can't be a good teacher if you don't continue to be a good student. That doesn't just mean keeping up with the latest guidelines from your governing body. It means questioning both the old basics and the new guidelines.

Most patients believe the longer a doctor practices, the better he gets. However, you and I both know that isn't necessarily true, don't we? Only when a doctor continues to read, study, and think can this be true. The minute you stop having time to read, both in your specialty and outside of it, is the moment you start becoming less of a doctor. Neither your patients nor your nurse will necessarily see any sign of your stagnation or deterioration, but you and I both know it's true. Doctors have no real way of receiving meaningful social or peer feedback, and this can make it hard to stay on the proper path. It's easy for a seasoned doctor to bluff, pontificate, and confabulate in a way that makes him seem very impressive to all who hear. It doesn't mean that he knows or remembers a damn thing.

There is often so much politics in medicine that being right can get you into trouble because the right ideas seem so radical or go against the current standard of practice. Please don't be part of this problem. Step away from that dark side and be part of the solution. I've respectfully included several suggestions for you, the seasoned and respected doctor.

Keep reading. If macular degeneration steals your vision, then learn braille. Doing your reading is a requirement at any level of medicine. No matter your age or career status, books and journals will occupy much of your time if you're doing things properly. The doctor who is nearing retirement owes it to his patients to keep reading right up until the last day.

Know the guidelines, but don't blindly follow them. I'll bet that two hundred years ago, the American Association of Leech Medicine published guidelines on all the uses of leeches in medicine. Every doctor had a copy of these guidelines and followed them faithfully. If a doctor strayed from these peer-reviewed guidelines, he would be censored or chastised by the powers that be.

Does that example sound ridiculous to you? Well, let's change the variables a little. Let's change the name of the association and the name of the treatment. The American Heart Association published guidelines on the use of statins in medicine. Every doctor had a copy of these guidelines and followed them faithfully. If a doctor strayed from these peer-reviewed guidelines, he would be censored or chastised by the powers that be. Same story, different players. The problem is that both these treatments, leeches and statins, were ill-conceived and continued to be *standard of care* long after it was clear that their use was foolish. They both offered little benefit to the average patient and were fraught with dangerous side effects.

The lesson here is to stay up to date with the guidelines but don't follow them blindly. The statin fiasco didn't have to last decades; it could have been killed quickly if doctors had kept examining the research and asking questions. Millions of patients have suffered, and billions of dollars have been spent on a class of drugs that effectively did nothing positive for the average patient. This should get you thinking: What else are you prescribing that is ill-advised? Always be thinking and exploring the literature.

Your patients love and trust you; you owe it to them to be right most of the time. I have always thought of my patients as my children, although some people frown on this outlook. It helps me and the way my mind works to have this perspective, but it also holds me to a very high standard. For example, if the AHA says that the newest Big Pharma pill will lower the risk of something, but when you read the actual research, it's obvious that the right people at the FDA were treated to the right lunches, and that special treatment affected the outcome of the recommendation. What should you do? If you don't hold your patient in a special place in your heart (even the difficult patients), then you might say, "Hey, who am I to question the big dogs? I'm just a small-town doc, trying to get by."

This rationalization might seem justified to you; however, it is one of the most shameful abdications of your position you could ever perform. Yes, you're between a rock and a hard place. Yes, there might be ramifications if you don't follow the guidelines. So what will you do? Thinking of my patients as my children makes it easy for me to tell the regulatory agencies to stick their guidelines up their... Well, I'll just say it makes it easy for me not to give my patient a pill fraught with side effects just because the big dogs said I should. I wouldn't do that to one of my children, and I won't do it to one of my patients either.

Dear colleague, read, think, teach, and heal. Be a part of the renaissance of modern medicine, not a part of its demise.

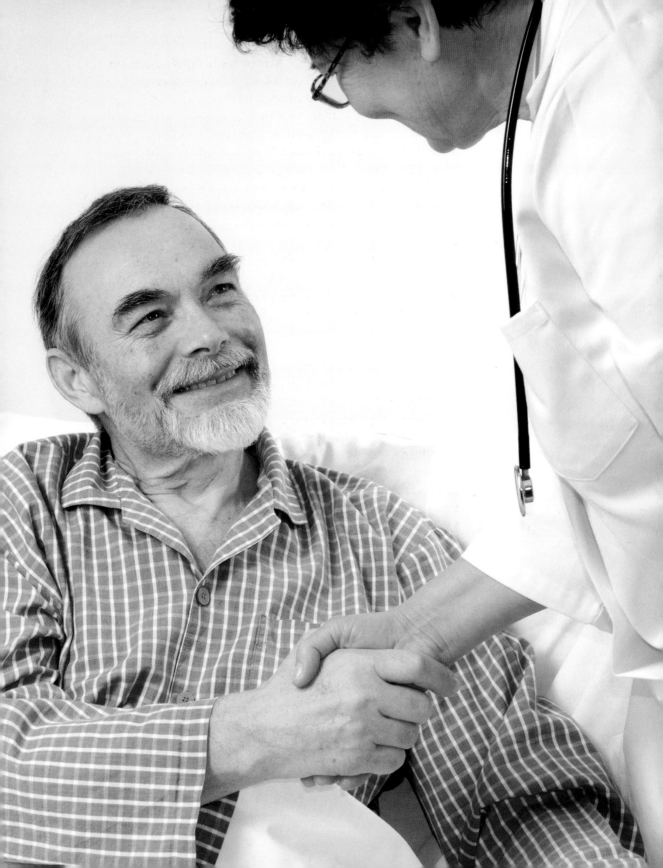

EPILOGUE

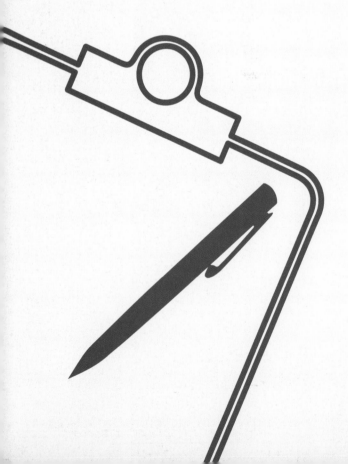

> ## "
> # Here's good advice for going into practice: go into partnership with nature; she does more than half the work and asks none of the fee.
>
> —Martin H. Fischer
> ## "

Congratulations. You have finished a book that was meant to change the way you think about your body, mind, and health. I hope you enjoyed it and learned a little something in the process. You must be wondering, "What should I do now?" Here are a few suggestions.

Do your homework.

At the end of each chapter, I named a book or website (or two) that I find to be useful for helping patients understand the concepts of the subject. Go back to the chapters that were most relevant to you and look for the homework sections. You will find that while doing your homework, you will come up with a unique plan for your health. It's up to you to decide which chapters are most important to you, and which homework assignments will help you most.

Decide whether you will keep your doctor.

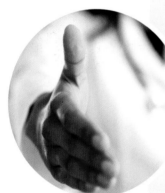

Will you try to train the doctor you have now, or do you need to find a new doctor? This might be a very hard decision. You don't have to decide right now. A good way to help you decide is to take this book, or some pages from your homework, to your next appointment to see how your doctor reacts. If he's willing to listen and work with you, then he may be a keeper. Doctors can change, just like anyone else can. (Remember, I used to be a regular doctor who recommended a low-fat, whole-grain diet and prescribed statins left and right.) If, however, he reacts negatively and doesn't seem interested, then it might be time to do some doctor shopping. Finding a doctor who will be your partner in health is a priceless thing.

Start applying what you have learned to your life and the lives of your loved ones.

Every small improvement you make in your diet and lifestyle now can lead to huge rewards later. Stopping milk or having your testosterone checked can lead to more improvement in your life than you might imagine. Taking baby steps in the beginning is both expected and appropriate. You can take bigger steps as you grow in your newfound knowledge.

Take more responsibility for your health.

Keeping you healthy is neither your doctor's job nor your spouse's. It's *your* job, and you only get so many chances to work on it. You're made of what you eat, so eat the right stuff. Your brain is filled with the knowledge you put in it, so put in good stuff. Your life is filled with what you accumulate, so make sure you keep only what you really like.

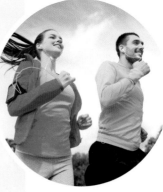

Enlist your family and friends.

Being healthy is so much easier when those closest to you are also striving for good health. If your spouse or best friend isn't on the right track, then share this book with them or gift them a copy. It won't take long before your work toward better health produces results that others can see. When people ask what you're doing, tell them and explain why you're doing it.

Join with me on a journey to improve your body, mind, and spirit.

Subscribe to my email newsletter. I'm not much of an email writer, so I promise not to bug you too much. I'll send occasional updates about new information, research, or books that I recommend. I also will alert you when my next book is released (if Neisha lets me write another one). I promise never to sell or give away any of your information or your email address. Subscribe at LMDTM@theberryclinic.com.

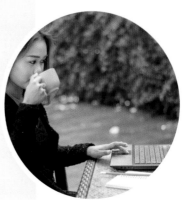

Word of mouth is crucial for any author to succeed. If you enjoyed this book, please consider leaving an honest review on Amazon.com, even if it's only a line or two. Writing a review is easy and takes just a minute. I would appreciate it greatly because it helps so much to get the message to others.

Join me on social media, and let's change the world.
There is no easier way to share good health info with the people you love than on social media. Sharing helpful info you have found on Facebook or Instagram is the new word of mouth. Together, we can make the world a healthier place. You can join me in the following places:

- ▶ YouTube: www.youtube.com/kendberrymd
- f Facebook: www.facebook.com/kendberry.md
- ⓘ Instagram: www.instagram.com/kendberry.md
- 🐦 Twitter: @KenDBerryMD
- ❘● Patreon: www.patreon.com/kendberrymd
- ⚡ Cameo: www.cameo.com/kendberry.md

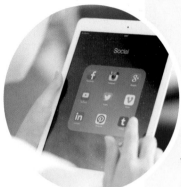

Thank you so much for giving my book a chance, and I wish you the very best in health.

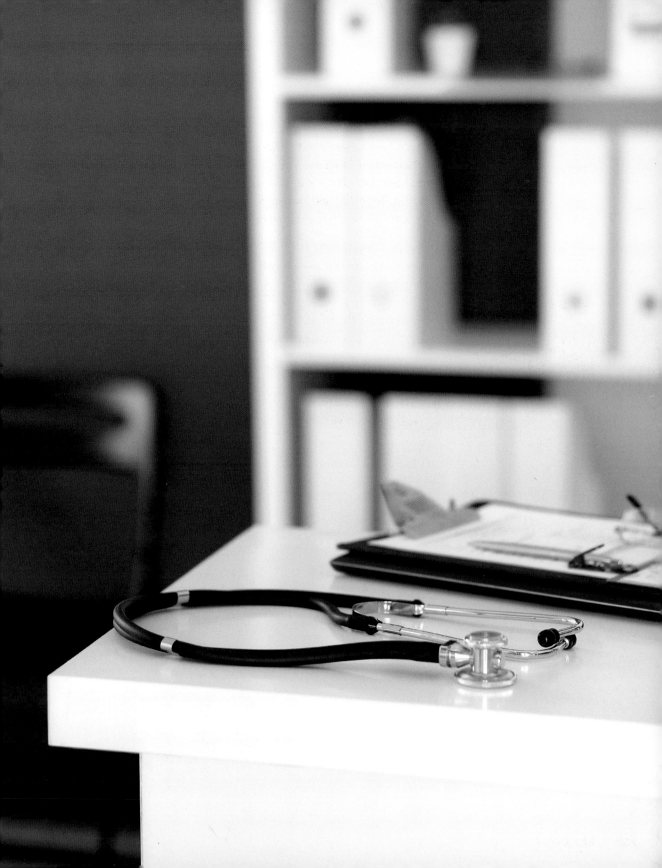

Index